SpringerBriefs in Psychology

For further volumes:
http://www.springer.com/series/10143

Kimberly Collica

Female Prisoners, AIDS, and Peer Programs

How Female Offenders Transform Their Lives

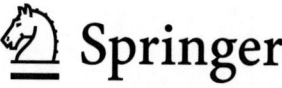 Springer

Kimberly Collica
Justice Studies
Berkeley College
Woodland Park, NJ, USA

ISSN 2192-8363   ISSN 2192-8371 (electronic)
ISBN 978-1-4614-5109-9   ISBN 978-1-4614-5110-5 (eBook)
DOI 10.1007/978-1-4614-5110-5
Springer New York Heidelberg Dordrecht London

Library of Congress Control Number: 2012945305

Printed on acid-free paper

Springer is part of Springer Science+Business Media (www.springer.com)

Preface

I became very interested in the topic of HIV and women in prison in 1999 when I began working at Taconic Correctional Facility coordinating their HIV prison-based peer program. The inmates had a tremendous interest in the program and we always had a tremendously positive response to every new program initiative. It seemed obvious that program participants were gaining an incredible amount of knowledge from being a part of CARE, but there was very little research on the subject area. To avoid a conflict of interest by studying the CARE Program, I decided to focus my study on ACE, which was across the street at Bedford Hills Correctional Facility. The results of the first study were quite promising and provided evidence that HIV prison-based peer programs do increase levels of knowledge about HIV/AIDS. As I progressed in my position, I also noticed that these programs had great benefits for the peers themselves. The women who worked for ACE/CARE were extremely successful and very well respected by prison staff and other inmates for their work. Disciplinary infractions decreased substantially for many of the women after they began working in these programs. I noticed increases in self-esteem and levels of confidence. I also noticed that when the women were finally eligible for release, they were able to obtain paid positions in the field of HIV. Most of these women who left never returned to prison, which made me consider the fact that these programs were not just about education, they were about redirection. There is little research on the effects of peer programs on the peers themselves. This factor, in combination with my interest in the success of ACE/CARE peers, led to further study on the issue of HIV programs.

The purpose of this book is to provide an overview of female incarceration and illustrate the benefits derived by female inmates who work in an HIV prison-based peer program, while adding to the criminology literature on female patterns of criminality and rehabilitation. It will provide a more in-depth understanding of how prison programs affect the processes of criminal desistance and behavioral changes for female inmates. Women involved in such programming have developed strong social bonds and high levels of self-esteem. These factors contributed to reduced levels of recidivism and institutional disciplinary infractions.

This book is framed within the broader perspective of women, HIV, and incarceration. Little research has been conducted on less traditional vocational opportunities behind bars, like HIV/AIDS peer education programs, particularly if such programs impact rehabilitative outcomes and reintegrative measures for the formerly incarcerated. These programs have not been given the attention they deserve in the literature. Researchers have discussed the overall benefits of HIV programming but rarely discuss the beneficial effects of such programming on the peers themselves. When benefits were cited, most researchers relied on anecdotal evidence.

It is evident that HIV peer programs are able to provide numerous benefits to prison officials by affording inmates with increased knowledge, accurate risk perceptions, a cost-effective method of providing educational services, etc. However, the effects transcend the benefits discussed in a majority of these studies. The pains of imprisonment for women can be improved by revolutionizing the way we view nontraditional programming in prison. A systematic research project has yet to be completed focusing on whether or not there is more to gain than knowledge and behavior change from these programs. In lieu of the limited programming available to female offenders, the evaluation of existing programs should be a foremost concern among correctional researchers, advocates, and administrators. This book offers an initial evaluation.

Woodland Park, NJ, USA   Kimberly Collica

Author Biography

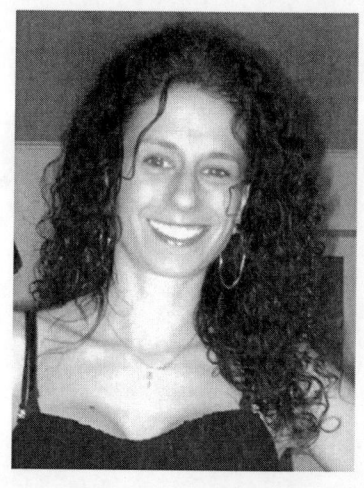

Dr. Kimberly Collica is a Professor of the Justice Studies Department and the Online Chairperson of the School of Professional Studies at Berkeley College. Prior to teaching, she worked for a women's correctional facility in New York State coordinating an HIV prison-based peer education program. She also worked for the Westchester County Department of Correction supervising their jail-based transitional services unit. She has extensive experience working with correctional populations and has over ten years of teaching and training experience in this area. Dr. Collica serves as a TOT (Train the Trainers) for the NYS Department of Health/AIDS Institute and is responsible for training professionals in HIV-related issues in the NYS Metropolitan area. Dr. Collica has a Ph.D. in Criminal Justice from the Graduate School and University Center of the City University of New York, an M.Phil. from the Graduate School and University Center, an MA in Criminal Justice from John Jay College, and a BA in Criminology from John Jay College. Her research focuses on female inmates, rehabilitation, reintegration, and issues surrounding HIV prison-based peer programming.

Acknowledgements

I would like to thank my friend, Joyce Lopez, for encouraging me to submit this book proposal. I would like to thank Sharon Panulla, Executive Editor, Sylvana Ruggirello, and Dr. Larry Sullivan for his comments and wisdom on the initial proposal. Editorial Assistant, Dhivya Chandraprathan, Project Manager, and Priyaa H Menon, Production Editor of Springer Science+Business Media, for their hard work and dedication toward the completion of this project. I would like to thank the New York State Department of Corrections and Community Supervision, particularly Elaine Humphrey, Program Research Specialist, and Paul Korotkin, Assistant Director of Research, for allowing me to conduct this study. I am tremendously grateful to all of the women of ACE and CARE, present and past, who spoke so openly and honestly with me. I have learned so much about myself and about life by working with them. I praise and admire them for their diligence in fighting the AIDS epidemic among women. I would like to thank my grandmother, Antoinette Taylor, my great friends, Carol Mendoza, Lisa Foreman, Karyn Albino, Patricia Chong, David Chong, Eric Grossman, Adam Welsh, Wilford Pinkney, Dr. Fein and Nory Padilla for always being so proud of me. I would also like to thank my two faithful companions: Jenny and Dominic, who were always by my side when I worked. Last, I would like to thank my family: my husband, Thomas Cox, my grandfather, Stanley Taylor, my doctoral twin, Dr. Gennifer Furst, my daughter, Annalise Cox (who was born just as I began writing this book and is my daily dose of joy), my stepsons (Dezmond, Dakota, and Ryan Cox my protector), my sisters (Elizabeth Collica, Katherine Varrin and Donna Collica) my brother and best friend, Anthony Collica, and my mom, Antoinette Varrin. I would especially like to thank my daughter, Antoinette Collica, who has served as my motivation for 19 years and continues to serve as my inspiration. You will always be my heart. I love you.

I would like to dedicate this book to my husband, Thomas Cox, who is always in my thoughts and my heart personally and professionally - "Don't let the name fool you."

Contents

Contents

Chapter 1
Women, Prison and, HIV: An Introduction

Introduction

The AIDS epidemic and the increase in incarceration for women are two major social phenomena that have had the most devastating and far reaching social effects on Americans in the last generation. Both caused considerable damage to the social fabric of American society and continue to damage millions of those infected with HIV. HIV and prison are inextricably linked and education has proved to be the one constant that mitigates the spread of both HIV and crime.

History of the Female Offender

Women offenders are the most neglected population throughout the history of the criminal justice system. In many areas of the USA, at least until the end of the nineteenth century, females did not have their own correctional institutions (Rafter, 1989). Due to their smaller numbers and the fact that they were isolated in attics or in separate areas of men's prisons, these women were neglected, physically abused, sexually abused, given minimal food, minimal medical care, minimal programming, and forced to live in deplorable and overcrowded conditions (Dobash, Dobash, & Gutteridge, 1986; Feinman, 1983; Pollock-Byrne, 1990; Rafter, 1989). It was after the Civil War that reformatories for women emerged due to increased concern surrounding the female offenders' conditions of imprisonment (Dobash et al., 1986). Race played a large role; these reformatories were utilized mainly for white women (Rafter, 1989). Black women were still confined to prisons and often subjected to the same harsh treatment as their male counterparts (Chesney-Lind, 1991).

The female reformatory opened a new career for female professionals in which social services could be provided to women by women. According to Schulz (1995), Female Quakers led the way by entering penal institutions to provide services and

K. Collica, *Female Prisoners, AIDS, and Peer Programs: How Female
Offenders Transform Their Lives*, SpringerBriefs in Psychology,
DOI 10.1007/978-1-4614-5110-5_1, © The Author 2013

serve as role models for female inmates. Sex scandals with male officers and harsh prison conditions allowed women of high social standing to successfully lobby for the creation of a female prison matron position. By the 1880s, states were establishing female-only prisons.

Early female pioneers of corrections were not interested in replacing men or in adopting traditional male models of law enforcement. By taking the concept of a *women's sphere* to a new level (i.e., just as they could clean houses, they could clean up the department of corrections), they were able to obtain gendered positions that were separate from men and, therefore, did not threaten men professionally (Schulz, 1995). Through the reformatory, it was believed that if women supervised other women, they would teach them how to be "good" and virtuous, which often meant learning how to become good wives and good mothers (Moyer, 1984; Rafter, 1989). Sadly, the domesticity skills provided to women in prison ignored their economic backgrounds and the fact that they needed to obtain employment upon release to support their families (Feinman, 1983). Female criminals were labeled as "fallen women" and considered to be morally degenerate (Dobash et al., 1986). "Many Americans believed that women offenders were born pure but had fallen, and thus were more depraved than male offenders. Because they deemed fallen women, unlike men, to be totally vile, lost and socially unredeemable, Americans treated female offenders more harshly than men" (Feinman, 1983, p. 14).

By the 1930s, both the reformatory and the other correctional institutions for women merged to form the women's prison system (Rafter, 1989). These institutions changed dramatically and were no longer run by women for women. "Rather, they supported the male-dominated prison system and adopted its values of isolation as well as traditional methods of prison discipline and inmate control" (Moyer, 1984, p. 48).

Female Incarceration Today

Today, there are many states without female-only correctional facilities; other states have only one female prison (Pollock-Byrne, 1990), which means that there are no specialized security classifications among female inmates (Rafter, 1989). All of the women, regardless of security level, are housed together. Unlike male inmates, if they experience problems while incarcerated (i.e., problems with another inmate or staff person), or would like to be closer to their family to encourage visitation, they either have limited options for transfer, or in states that only have one female facility, they have no options at all.

There are substantially more men than women in prison but this should not overshadow female incarceration rates, which have soared within the last decade, a consequence of the War on Drugs and subsequent sentencing reforms (i.e., mandatory minimum sentencing) (Chesney-Lind, 1991). Although female rates of incarceration have changed, the types of crimes women commit remain invariable. Most of the crime committed by female offenders is economically motivated and nonviolent (Pollock-Byrne, 1990). About one-third of females are serving time for a drug-related offense (Gondles, 1998). Unlike male offenders, many of these women are the sole supporters of their children and they suffer from a history of sexual and physical abuse, drug addiction, and prostitution (Chesney-Lind & Rodriguez, 1983).

Female offenders differ from their male counterparts in many other ways upon being admitted to prison. They are less likely than men to have a prior criminal record, to have committed a violent crime and to have returned to prison on a new charge or on a parole violation (Pollock-Byrne, 1990). These differences among female and male offenders appear to emerge in adolescence. When looking toward young offenders, juvenile girls are more likely than boys to be arrested for *status offenses* (i.e., illegal acts due to one's age). Hence, the juvenile justice system has been accused of criminalizing the survival strategies of many young girls who often runaway to escape abuse. Once on the streets, they are forced to engage in criminal and/or deviant behavior to survive (Chesney-Lind, 1989). Instead of helping them, we arrest them and label them as criminals.

Young white girls have historically been subjected to formal mechanisms of control when their sexual behavior violated conventional female norms (even as victims of sexual abuse), subjecting them to harsh and humiliating punishments inside of the courtroom and inside of the reformatory, while the sexual exploitation of young African-American girls continued to be ignored (Odem, 1995). The fact that these young girls were often victims of sexual abuse by their own family members went unnoticed, and in an attempt to maintain their daughters' purity, parents willingly turned their daughters over to the state (Odem, 1995). These girls were treated and labeled as criminally deviant in a system that blatantly ignored issues of class, race, gender, and victimization. The formal systems of social control played a large part "in labeling and shaping the crime problem" and their role in this process "is frequently underestimated" (Chesney-Lind, 1986, p. 78).

Incarceration Statistics for Female Offenders

Today, approximately seven million people in the USA are under some form of correctional supervision, with over two million incarcerated in the federal/state prison and city/county jail systems (BJS, 2012). Between 1978 and 1998, our inmate population tripled (Butterfield, 1995; Lawrence, Meors, Dubin, & Travis, 2002). Inmates are serving much longer sentences than ever before (Butterfield 1995). Surpassing South Africa, our country earned the title for incarcerating the most prisoners per capita in the world (Lewis, 1994), with 470 inmates per 100,000 American residents serving time behind bars (BJS, 2012). Prison is an expensive endeavor. On average, it costs taxpayers $31,307 per inmate per year, ranging from $14,603 in Kentucky to $60,076 in New York (Henrichson & Delaney, 2012). This price includes the direct costs of incarceration (i.e., health care, personnel, benefits, etc.), but fails to include the collateral costs such as social services, public assistance, and the financial strain placed upon families when a loved one is removed from the home (Henrichson & Delaney, 2012).

One out of every 31 persons is under some form of correctional supervision in the USA. For females, it is one out of every 89 women (Women in Prison Project, 2009). According to the National Criminal Justice Reference Services (NCJRS) (2011), 25.5% of all arrests yearly (13,120,947) were women, with 14.5% of such arrests occurring for female minors. Women comprise almost 10% of the USA's incarcerated jail/prison population. Of all state and federal female inmates, most are white (49%), followed by African-Americans (28%), and Latinas (17%) (Women In Prison Project, 2009). Racial disparities within our prison system are apparent. African-American women are 4.5 times more likely than white women and 2.5 times more likely than Latina women to be incarcerated. Latina women are 1.6 times more likely to be incarcerated than their white counterparts (Women In Prison Project, 2009).

When compared to men, the rates of incarceration for women are growing at a faster pace (5% vs. 3.3% per year, respectively). From 1995 to 2008, female incarceration increased by 203% (Women in Prison Project, 2009). Concomitantly, the number of women under parole and probation supervision has increased steadily since 1995. One out of every eight parolees and one out of every four probationers are females. According to the BJS (Bureau of Justice Statistics, 2012), 67% of releases will be returned to prison within a 3-year period. Women comprise 8.7% of such releases and 57.6% will be rearrested within 3 years of their release. Of those arrested, 39.9% are found guilty of their charge(s).

Inmate Differences by Gender

The experiences of incarcerated women and their backgrounds vary from that of their male counterparts. Contrary to popular belief, most women are not incarcerated for committing violent crimes. The proliferation of female incarceration is due to an increase in drug arrests and the implementation of mandatory sentencing laws.[1] Arrest rates may be on the rise but women are not becoming more violent. News stories report that index crimes, found in the FBI's Uniform Crime Report, for women, have increased. Most index crimes are associated with violence. However, index crimes include the crime of *larceny*. The crime of larceny is to blame for the increase, not violent behavior.

---

[1] Mandatory sentencing laws remove judicial discretion. In New York, the Rockefeller Drug Laws were largely responsible for the increase in female incarceration. Under the original legislation, offenders could receive 15 years to life for drug possession. Mitigating factors, such as abuse, could not be taken into account during sentencing.

The majority of women are in jail/prison for drug, property, or public order crimes. Only 14% of violent crimes are committed by women, with 75% of these violent crimes consisting of simple assault. Twenty-eight percent of those violent acts were committed by female minors (Greenfeld & Snell, 2000). In most instances (75%), females victimized other females. When violence was perpetrated against men, 35% of such cases involved an intimate partner. Most women offenders (62%) knew their victim. Homicide by women, directed mostly toward an intimate partner or family member (60% of cases), decreased steadily since 1993. Women who kill are much less likely than men who kill to have a criminal history and they are more likely to have killed as a result of domestic violence.

When involved in criminal activity, women often play an ancillary role to men. Even in the drug market, women occupy the lowest levels of the economic drug ladder (serving as lookouts, steerers,[2] or sellers). Since they are on the street, they are more visible to law enforcement and are more likely to be arrested (Maher, 2000). Their low criminal status precludes them from obtaining information on "higher-ups" which might help them obtain a plea bargain.

The incarceration of women affects minor children more than the incarceration of men. Seventy-five percent of incarcerated women have a minor child; 64% report living with their minor child/children prior to arrest (Greenfeld & Snell, 2000; Snell & Morton, 1994; Women in Prison Project, 2009). When men are incarcerated, most minor children reside with the mother. Over half of the children of incarcerated mothers are living with the grandparents, 10% are in foster care, and the rest are residing with other family members or friends. When women are incarcerated, children are displaced.

Financially, most female offenders have inconsistent to no employment history prior to their arrest. Thirty-seven percent of women earned less than $600 per month before their arrest and 30% reported dependence upon public assistance (Travis, Solomon, & Waul, 2001). Women are more likely than men to have mental illness, poorer physical health, and a history of physical/sexual abuse. Although both male and female inmates experienced high rates of abuse as children, the cycle of abuse for females continues to permeate their adolescence and adulthood.

Many female offenders reported drug and alcohol problems. Over one-half of female offenders used alcohol/drugs at the time of their crime. Only 1% of women were identified as chronic recidivists, whereas 6% of male offenders were believed to be chronic adult criminal offenders (Wolfgang, Figilio, & Sellin, 1972). On average, females received shorter sentences than male inmates for every charge except for property offenses. In terms of prison admissions, they comprised 10% of those committed for negligent manslaughter, 11% for larceny, 12% for arson, 31% for fraud, 14% for drug possession, 11% for drug trafficking, and 1% for sexual assault. On average, when dealing with the female offender, we are dealing with a nonviolent person (Greenfeld & Snell, 2000).

---

[2] A steerer is one who "steers" or directs a user to a place/person to obtain drugs. It is one of the lowest possible positions held in the drug market.

Statistics on Women Offenders and HIV

Since the 1980s, over 619,000 Americans died from AIDS-related complications (AIDS.gov, 2012). As many as one million Americans are currently infected with HIV (Sternberg, 2004) and about one-third of these individuals do not know that they are infected (CDC, 2001). Furthermore, it is estimated that there are over 40,000 new cases of HIV infection nationally every year (CDC 2001; Holmberg, 1996), disproportionately affecting minority populations. There is also concern that HIV rates may be rising in the USA for the first time in years (Sternberg, 2004).

According to the Center for Disease Control (CDC) (1999), African-Americans are six times more likely and Hispanics are three times more likely to test positive for HIV when compared to whites. African-Americans and Hispanics represent 61% of all AIDS cases (CDC, 2001). In combination, African-American and Hispanic women represent less than one-fourth of the US female population, but they comprise three-fourths of the total number of AIDS cases for women in this country since 1981. Indeed, AIDS is the leading cause of death among African-American women, between the ages of 25 and 44 years, and it is one of the leading causes of death for women overall in this age range. Women are the fastest growing population acquiring this infection. From 1989 to 1999, the rate of HIV infection tripled for women and female adolescents, with heterosexual sex as their most common mode of transmission (75% of new cases) (JAMA HIV/AIDS Information Center, 1999).

When we examine the rates of HIV infection among incarcerated populations, particularly females in New York State (NYS), the numbers are more confounding. Although HIV rates and AIDS diagnoses among prisoners have decreased since 1999 (Maruschak, 2002), prison populations are still disproportionately represented in the HIV epidemic. Overall, 2.2% of state inmates and .8% of federal inmates are known to be HIV positive, and by the end of 2000, 5,528 of these inmates were diagnosed with AIDS (Maruschak, 2002).

At the time of this research, NYS had 70 prisons with approximately 70,000 inmates (3,000 were females) (Goord, 2001). Currently, NYS has 67 prisons with 56,000 offenders; less than 3,000 (approximately 4% of the prison population) are female (NYSDOCCS, 2012; 2008). The rate of AIDS cases among prisoners is six times higher than that of the general population (Hammett, Harmon, & Maruschak, 1999) and NYS reported the highest number of HIV positive inmates in the country (Hammett et. al., 1999; Lance-McCullough, Tesoriero, Sorin, & Stern, 1994). However, since 2002, the New York State Department of Corrections and Community Supervision (NYSDOCCS) reported tremendous decreases in cases of HIV infection and AIDS-related deaths (NYSDOCS, 2002). This may be related to improvements in HIV medications and treatments, an increase in the quality and quantity of HIV educational classes and an overall decrease in New York State's prison population.

Previously, blind studies in New York State prisons indicated that approximately 20% of female inmates tested positive for HIV compared to a 7% seroprevalence rate among NYS male inmates (Miki, 1998). Generally, female inmates have a higher rate of HIV infection than male inmates (Hammett et al., 1999). In the USA,

3.6% of all female inmates are known to be HIV infected, compared to a 2.2% seroprevalence rate among their male counterparts (Maruschak, 2002). Inmates are more likely to test positive for HIV infection if they were subsequently charged with a drug offense (Cotten-Oldenburg, Jordan, Martin, & Kupper, 1999; Hammett et al., 1999), if they were injectable drug users (IDU), if they traded sex for drugs (Harrison, Butzin, Inciardi, & Martin, 1998), and if they lived in NYC prior to their arrest (Lance-McCullough et al., 1994). The greatest number of AIDS cases related to IDU has been documented in the New York City Metropolitan Area (Des Jarlais & Friedman, 1988; NYSDOH, 2002), with 31% of AIDS cases in New York State credited to IDU (NYSDOH, 2002). Sexual abuse history plays a role in HIV infection for women. Women with a history of sexual abuse partake in more risky HIV-related behaviors (i.e., prostitution, sex with multiple partners, and unprotected sex) when compared to women who were not sexually abused (Mullings, Marquart, & Hartley, 2003).

Effects of Incarceration on Women

Criminal sanctions have "invisible punishments" or unintended consequences (i.e., disenfranchisement, limitations on access to employment opportunities, public housing, public assistance, or federal/state aid for college programming, termination of parental rights, etc.) (see Travis, 2002). Although the restoration of rights is a contentious issue, it is a formidable hindrance to the formerly incarcerated. When denied the ability to live in public housing or denied access to certain employment opportunities, the formerly incarcerated are left with few avenues to successfully pursue rehabilitative goals.

Housing tends to be the foremost concern for both female and male releases (Lanier & Paoline, 2005). Without national data on the incidence of those with felony records excluded from public housing, it is difficult to know how many people are affected. According to a report by the Human Rights Watch (2004), it is estimated that this number exceeds several million people. Considering that those leaving American correctional facilities will have few housing options available to them upon release, public safety is a primary concern. These policies, enacted by the federal government, known as "one strike policies," are "arbitrary and unreasonably overbroad" (Human Rights Watch, 2004, p. 3). Poor people and people of color are disproportionately represented in our prison population, thereby disproportionately discriminated against by these federal regulations. Such regulations allow the Public Housing Authority to deny housing applications to prospective tenants on the basis of a prior felony conviction, regardless of how much time has passed since its occurrence. If an offender has family members who live in public housing, he/she will be prohibited from residing with them, leaving the homeless shelter as his/her only option.

These policies doubly marginalize women leaving prison, many of whom are trying to reestablish ties with their children (if they did not lose custody of their children while incarcerated). With the passage of FASA (Federal Adoption Assistance and Child Welfare Reform Act) in 1980, if a child is placed in foster care for 18–22 months, the state can begin parental termination procedures. "Although this legislation was meant to avoid multiple short-term placements that worsen the disruption for children, parents with sentences that exceed the allowable time may be unable to comply with reunification requirements before or after release" (Reed & Reed, 2004, p. 264). Due to multiple foster home placements, incarcerated women who have children in the foster care system face enormous difficulty in locating and maintaining contact with their children. Even if they know the location of their children, the distance between the children's residence and the prison inhibits the ability to visit often (Reed & Reed, 2004). Upon release, women face additional barriers to family reunification. Most women are unable to acquire decent housing if they do not have custody of their children and many cannot regain custody of their children until they have adequate housing. Due to "one strike policies," they will most likely be denied the ability to reside in public housing and they will most likely be unable to afford unsubsidized housing. Regrettably, many women may be forced to return to unsatisfactory living conditions (i.e., living with a former abuser) (Human Rights Watch, 2004).

According to the Human Rights Watch (2004), offenders should not be penalized by these laws, particularly after 5 years of release, when the rate of recidivism after this time is exceptionally low. "Periods of exclusion beyond 5 years, especially lifetime exclusions, make little sense in light of this reality" (p. 35). In lieu of this evidence, these harsh sentencing reforms, which last a lifetime, appear to be yet another example of bad criminal justice policy.

If an ex-offender does not recidivate, his/her criminal record will continue to follow him/her forever and will remain a continuous impediment to successful reintegration, particularly in obtaining employment. Without the ability to obtain modest housing, the chances of obtaining decent employment decrease substantially. Offenders can interview for an employment position but prospective employers cannot contact them if they do not have an address or telephone number. It is apparent that housing serves as an important link to employment opportunity and maintenance.

With this is mind, it becomes even more important to provide offenders with employment skills that can actually help them to obtain stable jobs once released. Ideally, this process should begin months, even years, before offenders are released back into the community. Jobs that inmates have while incarcerated are often geared toward maintaining the day-to-day operations of the facility (i.e., porters). These jobs are necessary to maintain facility operations but have little utility in the outside world. In order for inmates to be successful once released, they need to possess job skills that will allow them to earn a decent wage to diminish the likelihood of relapse and recidivism. This is particularly important for female offenders. "Women offenders are often involved in codependent relationships that stimulate their criminal activities. Skills are important for women so that they also gain social independence, thus removing them from codependent relationships and other circumstances that contribute to their criminal lifestyles" (Koons, Burrow,

Morash, & Bynum, 1997, p. 528). Furthermore, most jobs and training programs in female facilities are traditionally gender based (i.e., cooking, secretarial, etc.). Such jobs, upon release, pay very little.

Effects of Incarceration on HIV

According to the NYSDOH AIDS Institute (2008), many HIV positive inmates receive health care for the first time in a long time as a result of their incarceration. Incarceration allows for health-care interventions and counseling, much of which is nonexistent while offenders are living on the streets. Although some argue that prison does not avail itself to preeminent health care, it may be the only health care an offender has received in years; this proves to be especially true for the female offender who has most likely neglected her gynecological needs. Such health care is imperative in the successful treatment of HIV and other underlying health conditions.

Not all inmates are aware of their HIV status. HIV testing policies in prison vary according to jurisdiction and can include voluntary testing policies (inmates can choose whether or not they want an HIV test), routine testing policies (inmates are routinely tested for HIV but have the right to refuse testing), and mandatory testing policies (inmates have no choice as to whether they are tested for HIV) (Brinkley-Rubenstein & Cornett, 2010). Eighteen state systems and the federal system sub-scribe to mandatory testing (Brinkley-Rubenstein & Cornett, 2010). Mandatory policies prevent an inmate from making decisions regarding his/her health and they assume that the offender is emotionally prepared to handle a positive test result.

Depending on the correctional system, inmates with HIV may be segregated from general population, such as in South Carolina or Alabama (Edwards, 2010). These policies discriminate against offenders with HIV. By segregating them in special units, their HIV status is inadvertently disclosed. Segregation hinders reha-bilitation; these inmates are prohibited from working or attending educational/voca-tional classes or programs. The inability to engage in specific programming while incarcerated can affect their ability to obtain early release, especially via the parole board. In addition, these inmates are typically housed in maximum security facili-ties, irrespective of their crime, at a tremendous cost to taxpayers (Edwards, 2010).

Incarcerated offenders do not have the means to protect against HIV if they are engaging in risky behaviors behind bars, such as needle use for drugs or tattooing or unprotected sexual activity, whether consensual or coerced. None of the correc-tional systems in the USA provide clean needles or materials to clean needles (i.e., bleach). Condom distribution is available in some larger metropolitan jails (i.e., NYC, San Francisco, LA, Philadelphia, and Washington, DC); only two state sys-tems (Vermont and Mississippi) provide condoms on a limited basis (Dolan, Lowe, & Shearer, 2004; NYSDOH AIDS Institute, 2008).

Most inmates know their HIV status prior to incarceration (NYSDOH AIDS Institute, 2008). Inmates housed in non-mandatory testing systems may keep their status a secret and opt to forgo treatment during incarceration to reduce stigma. Inmates receiving HIV medications often have to stand on long med lines in the morning to receive their antiviral therapy. In facilities where many originate from the same neighborhoods and lineage, it is better to decline treatment rather than risk having someone they know discover their HIV status.

Incarceration is highly stressful. Offenders are worried about their families and their own well-being. Stress can negatively affect one's health, especially if they present with a compromised immune system, as in the case with HIV. Prison-related stress affects CD4[3] counts; incarcerated persons are more likely to have lowered T-cell counts when compared to members of the general HIV-infected community (Griffin, Ryan, Briscoe, & Shadle, 1996).

The dependency upon the correctional system can make the return to the community more difficult and the treatment of HIV more complicated. The longer one is incarcerated, the more dependent they become. After being told when to wake up, when to take their medicine, when to eat, and when to go to the bathroom, for a period of many years, we preclude offenders from making any "real" decisions while incarcerated. At the conclusion of this period, we release them with $30 in "gate money," a bus/train ticket and tell them to make all of the right decisions. It is often difficult, particularly with all of the stressors faced upon release (i.e., employment, housing, family issues, addiction issues, etc.), and the lack of practice while imprisoned, to make "good" decisions, least of all to maintain treatment adherence.

ACE and CARE

One way to mitigate the negative impact of HIV on incarceration is to implement and maintain HIV prison-based peer education programs. These programs are cost effective, provide an invaluable service to correctional administrators, and can serve as rehabilitative and reintegrative tools for inmate peers. Jobs in the field of HIV can offer women the opportunity to support themselves and their family. Teaching and counseling skills developed within the correctional setting have utility in the community. Once these skills are honed and experience is gained, paid positions in the HIV field with community-based organizations are possible. Evidence on the effectiveness of such programs is based upon two well-established prison-based peer programs: The ACE and CARE Programs in NYS.

---

[3] CD4 or T-cells are the coordinators of the immune system. They are responsible for instructing the B-cell to produce antibodies to certain antigens. When T-cells are destroyed by HIV, immune function is severely compromised. Those with a T-cell count below 200 or those who present with an opportunistic infection (i.e., an infection, such as hepatitis, toxoplasmosis, or cervical cancer, which takes the opportunity to enter the body when the immune system is already comprised) are diagnosed with AIDS.

The ACE Program at Bedford Hills Correctional Facility

The ACE (AIDS, Counseling and Education) Program is located at Bedford Hills Correctional Facility (BHCF), which houses approximately 792 female inmates, serving as a reception center for all female inmates entering state prison in NY (NYSDOCS, 2003). According to former Superintendent Elaine Lord (1995), each year there are 3,000 women who pass through Bedford's reception area.[4] They will either remain at Bedford or they will be "drafted" (sent) to another facility. Most of the women incarcerated at Bedford have "6 or more years to serve on their minimum sentences before they can even appear before the parole board for release consideration (p. 257)." The average time of incarceration is approximately eight and one-third years, and one out of every five women entering the NYS system of corrections is HIV positive. Programs are an important facet of the facility but they will always take second place to security. "Security takes precedence over all other functions and absorbs the majority of the funding (p. 263)." With so many issues to account for, the ACE program continues to strive to educate female inmates about HIV/AIDS.

Since its inception in 1985, ACE is one of the most widely recognized peer-led inmate programs in the world. ACE is contracted by the AIDS Institute/New York State Department of Health to provide HIV-related services for female inmates. Yearly, ACE renders HIV/AIDS education to approximately 3,000 women. In addition, the program provides individual counseling, HIV testing, outreach services, support groups, annual events, professional trainings, and discharge planning/case management.

ACE was created in response to the devastating effects of the AIDS epidemic on female inmates (ACE, 1998). In the mid-1980s, a handful of inmates were extremely concerned about the effect that AIDS was having on women prisoners, a disease that they knew very little about. After holding meetings in the yard or on the walkways, the women of BHCF decided that they wanted to start a formal HIV program. Initially the program began through the efforts of five female inmates who submitted a proposal to the superintendent (Act Up/NY, 1990). After many trials and tribulations, and with the support and guidance of their Superintendent, Elaine Lord, the women were allowed to enact ACE. This was the first program of its kind and created concerns among prison officials; allowing inmates to manage their own program might create a disproportionate amount of power in the hands of those that the prison staff was trying to manage and control. In the beginning, volunteers came up to the facility to train the women to provide education to their peers. This continued until the services were eventually contracted to an outside agency through the AIDS Institute.

The women are trained to provide a ten-session workshop, entitled "Community Prep," which is delivered over the course of 2 weeks, 3 h/day during the first few weeks that a woman is at BHCF. Topics include (a) stigma, (b) what is HIV/

---

[4] All information regarding BHCF, TCF, and ACE/CARE programs is accurate for the time period when data were originally collected in 2005.

AIDS, (c) transmission, (d) testing and treatments, (e) nutrition and drug/alcohol awareness, (f) holistic and alternative treatments, (g) women's health issues, (h) video viewing and discussion, (i) self-esteem, and (j) review. Similar programming is also provided to women in ASAT (Alcohol, Substance Abuse, and Treatment Programming), IPC (in-patient care) (i.e., those with physical illness and ailments), ICP (Intermediary Care Program) (i.e., inmates who are segregated from general population as a result of a mental illness), and the nursery mothers living on the grounds of BHCF with their babies. ACE also has an ACE organization, which provides inmates from general population with membership privileges to the ACE Program. Although these women do not work for ACE as peers, they are invited to participate in an intensive workshop series, annual events, and some of them volunteer to provide HIV related services to the rest of population. The organization also consists of former ACE peers, who have moved on to other employment positions in the facility, but who do not wish to sever all ties with the program.

In addition to education, the ACE program provides support groups (an HIV-infected group, an HIV-affected group, and a cancer support group), outreach, counseling services, an annual barbecue for ACE organizational members, an AIDS quilt project, an annual AIDS Walk-a-thon (which raises money for an outside HIV/AIDS service provider), and an annual world AIDS Day (money raised from the walk-a-thon is given to a chosen HIV agency). Although no longer in existence, ACE employed a buddy system which allowed ACE peers to escort women to Bedford's hospital to help them understand the medical information provided by the doctors and nurses. Moreover, outside speakers are invited to the facility during the year to provide the women with health-related information or updated information on HIV and other vital health issues.

The CARE Program at Taconic Correctional Facility

The CARE (Counseling, AIDS, Resource, and Education) Program at TCF (Taconic Correctional Facility), educating approximately 600 women annually, is located directly across the street from BHCF. Since TCF is a medium security facility, holding approximately 400 inmates, many women at BHCF will pass through TCF before they are eventually released back into the community. This allows many women who worked at ACE to continue providing the same HIV services when drafted to TCF. Albion Correctional Facility, located near the Canadian border, approximately 10 h north of TCF and BHCF, is also a medium security facility for women. Albion has a HIV peer program called REACH, but unlike CARE and ACE, this program is sponsored by another community-based organization, Rural Opportunities. Although women employed by ACE or CARE may work for Reach if drafted up to Albion and vice versa, the Reach Program was not included in this study. Due to financial and time constraints and different management, it was not feasible for the author to travel to Albion Correctional Facility to interview these women.

According to the NYSDOCS (2003), TCF started as a reformatory for women in 1913 and was a satellite of BHCF. In 1973, TCF became a separate facility and was initially used to house male offenders. In 1989, the facility returned to housing female inmates and became the only CASAT (Comprehensive, Alcohol, Substance, Abuse, and Treatment Program) facility for women in NYS. CASAT is a 6-month, presumptive work release program. After the women complete their CASAT Program, they will be drafted to either Phoenix House in Brooklyn (a drug treatment community), Bayview Correctional Facility in Manhattan, or Albion Correctional Facility in Albion to begin a work release program. Slightly less than one-half of TCF's population is CASAT eligible, the rest are slated as general population.

CARE did not begin as an inmate initiative as it did in the prison across the street. Based on a growing concern from some female prisoners about the AIDS epidemic, the head of chaplain services, Sister Antonia McGuire (who provided HIV supportive services for male inmates at Taconic and Sing Sing Correctional Facility), wanted to start a program similar to ACE. She was approached by several inmates in the facility who asked her to help them create a program for women who were dying of AIDS-related complications. With problems of their own, ACE staff was unable or unwilling to help Sister Antonia begin a program at TCF. With Superintendent Charles Hernandez's permission (Former Superintendent of Taconic), she decided to start a program by herself in the beginning of 1989 and call it CARE. The support of his administration allowed the CARE Program to flourish at Taconic. Along with the help of outside volunteers, one group of inmates were trained to provide HIV counseling on the housing units in English and another group was trained to provide HIV counseling on the housing units in Spanish. CARE also implemented the buddy system. Buddies would help the women who were ill by cleaning their rooms, cooking for them, feeding them, playing games with them, or just keeping them company. Most importantly, they were allowed to accompany the women to the clinic. They would help the clients to understand the information that was being given to them by the doctors, and for the Spanish-speaking women, they had someone they could trust who would translate the doctor's information. Sister Antonia, managed the CARE Program until the end of 1989. It was during this year that the ACE and CARE Programs finally merged under one contract from the NYS AIDS Institute. An alliance that she had sought months earlier finally became a reality. This contract, which remains at $130,000 per year for both programs[5], was held by at least two different agencies until Women's Prison Association won the contract in 1992.

The women in CARE provide a 14-session workshop to inmates in CASAT, ASAT, the nursery, and Transitional Services (a reentry training program for mostly women in general population who will be returning home shortly or are slated to appear in front of the parole board for release consideration). Transitional Services Programming is provided in the school building for a period of 2 weeks, 3 h/day, and offered to women shortly before release, while the other programs are provided

---

[5] This information was correct when data was originally collected in 2005.

biweekly directly on the housing units for a period of 6 consecutive months. The topics are as follows: (a) what is HIV/AIDS and the immune system, (b) stigma and blame, (c) transmission, risky behaviors, and risk reduction, (d) methods of contraception, (e) self-esteem, (f) nutrition, (g) women's issues, (h) medications, (i) HIV testing and partner notification, (j) opportunistic infections, (k) reproductive anatomy and physiology, (l) sexually transmissible infections, (m) living with HIV/AIDS, and (n) video viewing and discussion.

In addition to education, inmate peers provide counseling, outreach services, and facilitate a women's issues support group. The CARE Office offers many other valuable programs such as the New York State Department of Health TOT (train the trainer) courses, which train the women as HIV community educators or HIV pre- and posttest counselors (this program is offered three times per year). There are bimonthly Health Education Days (a representative from an outside agency presents a workshop on a health-related topic besides HIV such as lupus, reproductive health, cancer, domestic violence, contraception, hepatitis, rape, and transgender issues), an AIDS Quilt Project, an Annual Health and Resource Fair (approximately 25 agencies from the community staff information tables and establish connections with those that will be released), an Annual AIDS Dance-a-thon (money is raised by the women to donate to an outside HIV service provider), and an Annual World AIDS Day (money raised by the women from the dance-a-thon is donated to an agency of their choice). For the last 6 years prior to this research, CARE donated the proceeds from the AIDS dance-a-thon to the Birch Camp, a camp that takes HIV-infected/affected children from New York City and their family to an upstate New York camp for 1 week during the summer. Birch is a program that is often praised by the female inmates. Some women, after release, have worked as volunteers for Camp Birch. In addition to the facility events, both CARE and ACE have a bilingual educator on staff and offer free information to inmate population in both English and Spanish.

The ACE/CARE Civilian Staff

ACE and CARE employ five civilians through WPA.[6] Unlike many other peer programs across the country, these civilians are based in the facility on a full-time basis. The supervisor of prison-based services oversees both the ACE and CARE programs, but her main office is located at BHCF. There is a CARE Coordinator and an ACE Coordinator; both are responsible for supervising and training the women in their respective facilities, as well as coordinating annual events, and training programs. The other two civilians, a test counselor and a discharge planner, provide services at both facilities. The HIV pre- and posttest counselor offers both anonymous and confidential testing in accordance with the New York State Department of Health,

---

[6] This number was accurate at the time data were collected. Due to dwindling AIDS funding, the program structure changed and there are fewer civilians employed.

and the discharge planner provides discharge planning services to women who are HIV positive. Because of ACE's and CARE's connection to Women's Prison Association, an agency that has been servicing the needs of ex-offenders since 1844, important follow-up services are provided when the women are released.

WPA offers women case management, education, counseling, a transitional residence for women who want to reunite with their minor children (Sarah Powell Huntington House), an alternative to incarceration program (Hopper Home), legal assistance for women who may have lost custody of their children (Incarcerated Mother's Law Project), housing placement, employment skills, parenting classes, supportive services, peer escorts, peer mentors, and prison and jail-based services. (Conly, 1998).[7] These services will help to ease a woman's transition back into the community. Unlike many other agencies in the NYC area that service the formerly incarcerated, WPA is gender specific and works exclusively with women who have criminal justice involvement.

Inmate Staff

At the time of this research, the CARE Office and the ACE Office each employed five peer workers. For employment eligibility, inmates must have a high school diploma or GED, a good disciplinary history and participate in the TOTs. Both programs are allocated one slot for women who do not currently possess their GED or high school diploma, as long as they are making progress toward their degree. For both offices, interested inmates must submit a resume to the program coordinator. If deemed suitable, the inmates will have their first interview with the coordinator. If the coordinator believes that the inmate would make a good candidate for employment, a second interview will be scheduled. During the second interview, the prospective worker will be interviewed by the entire peer staff and they will also be required to present a 5 to 10-min teaching demonstration. After the applicant leaves, the inmate staff and the coordinator will make a joint decision on whether or not to hire the individual. Since the inmates are very involved in the hiring of new peer staff persons, this makes both ACE/CARE extremely unique; it is doubtful that many prisons would be comfortable allowing inmates to be part of such a process. New staff is reviewed after 3 months. If they successfully complete their probationary period (most are successful), they become permanent peers. New peers will be given a policy and procedure manual. They are required to sign a confidentiality clause and they are trained and mentored by both the coordinator and inmate peers. Hiring for CARE and ACE is very methodical but it will prepare the women for the "real world's" interviewing process upon release. Since many of the peers never had legitimate employment before their incarceration, this process provides valuable interview

---

[7] Some of these programs were eliminated recently due to reduced funding.

experience. The ACE Office and CARE Office are open during regular business hours but the inmate staff is on call 24 h a day, 7 days a week.

Inmates in both programs serve as role models for the rest of inmate population. Continuous disciplinary infractions (i.e., being out of place, fighting, insubordination to security staff, etc.) will result in job termination and program reassignment. Although this job can provide the peers with important skills, it can also lead to high levels of stress. Their behavior is constantly monitored by staff. Any indiscretion could jeopardize their position or the program's credibility. The peers are called upon at all hours of the day to counsel and provide information, even when they are in the shower, taking a nap, or trying to exercise or eat. However, if they have the ability to provide services in this highly restrictive and highly stressful environment, they should be able to successfully provide these same services in the community.

Conclusion

HIV prison-based programming is a way to mitigate crime and HIV, especially for female offenders whose needs and issues are diverse and differ from those of male offenders. HIV peer programs are able to provide numerous benefits to prison officials by providing inmates with increased knowledge and accurate risk perceptions. They are a cost-effective method of providing educational services. Although many researchers have pointed to the beneficial effects of peer programs on the peers themselves, the evidence is anecdotal at best. This has led to a serious gap in the knowledge base surrounding peer education programs. The current study provides further evidence on the beneficial effects of HIV peer programs and assists in bridging the gap between prior research and current anecdotal evidence. Not every program will serve as a rehabilitative tool for every inmate, but HIV prison programming may further rehabilitative goals for a small sample of inmates, while providing a valuable service to the rest of general population. The way one adapts or does not adapt to the prison environment can directly impact the inmate's behavior and lead to increased disciplinary problems. These behavioral problems can affect an inmate's opportunity to reintegrate successfully back into her community upon release. The study conducted on ACE/CARE, two HIV prison-based peer programs, shows how these two unique programs can provide a positive form of adaptation for some inmates when they enter prison and still serve as a mechanism for support once these women are released. It serves as a tool to mitigate the problem of crime (by lessening recidivism) and HIV (by decreasing risky behavior).

Chapter 2
Crime Trajectories and Crime Desistance

Introduction

When we examine the behavior of habitual adult offenders, we want to know why they fail to "age out" of crime. For those who commit crime after the age of 25 but eventually discontinue, we also want to consider the factors that contribute to their desistance. What do these offenders have in common? It appears that the answer may lie in the foundations of Hirschi's (1969) social control theory. Social control theory maintains that individuals are likely to commit crime when their bonds to conventional society are deficient or damaged. Life course theory expands upon this explanation and not only discusses the importance of bonds to conventional society in modifying behaviors but also examines the quality and strength of these bonds. In accordance with life course theorists, there are certain life transitions that can modify lifelong trajectories. These transitions can contribute to a desire and an ability to desist from future criminal activities. It appears that the strength of the social bonds that develop from working as an HIV peer educator during incarceration will serve as a life transition that can alter the criminal trajectory, thus increasing levels of institutional and post-release success.

Life Course Theory

Sampson and Laub (1995) maintain that criminal behavior can change if the offender experiences "transitions or turning points [that] can modify life trajectories. They can redirect paths" (Sampson & Laub, 1992, p. 66; Sampson & Laub, 1995, p. 144). They state, "A trajectory is a pathway or line of development over the life course span such as worklife, marriage, parenthood, self-esteem or criminal behavior". Trajectories refer to long-term patterns and sequences of behavior, while "transitions are marked by specific life events that are embedded in trajectories and evolve

K. Collica, *Female Prisoners, AIDS, and Peer Programs: How Female Offenders Transform Their Lives*, SpringerBriefs in Psychology, DOI 10.1007/978-1-4614-5110-5_2, © The Author 2013

over shorter time spans" (p. 66). "Transitions are always embedded in trajectories that give them distinctive form and meaning (Elder, 1985, p. 31)." The period and sequence in which a transition occurs can affect the impact of the transition on future criminal trajectories. How transitions influence behavior modification will depend on one's capacity to adapt to abrupt or gradual changes in life trajectories. The same transition can manifest itself differently depending on the time period in which it occurs[1] and the way in which the offender responds to the situation (Benson, 2002). "The same event or transition followed by different adaptations can lead to different trajectories" (Sampson & Laub, 1992, p. 66).

Life course theory is guided by social control theory, which is not concerned with why people deviate from conventional behavior, but with why people conform to legal and social norms (Akers, 1997). Unlike many theories of criminal behavior, social control seeks to explain conformity, not deviancy. There is a need to explain why people conform, not why they deviate. It is primarily based on the Hobbessian notion that we are not born as conformists; we all have the ability to engage in criminal behavior (Wiatrowski, Griswold, & Roberts, 1981). The central thesis of social control theory is derived from Travis Hirschi's social bonding/control theory as stated in his book, *Causes of Delinquency* (1969). "Delinquent acts result when an individual's bond to society is weak or broken" (Hirschi, 1969, p. 16). Hirschi gave a more comprehensive explanation of criminal behavior when compared to previous control theorists. "Hirschi formulated a control theory that brought together elements from all previous control theories and offered new ways to account for delinquent behavior" (Akers, 1997, p. 85).

The four elements that characterize the social bond are *attachment, commitment, involvement,* and *belief.* Each element of the bond is interrelated but independently effects delinquency (Matsueda, 1982). First, the more *attached* we are to others and the more we value their opinions, the more likely we are to participate in conventional activity. Second, the more *commitment* we have to participating in conventional activity (the more time and energy we are willing to invest in conformity, particularly in terms of our educational and vocational aspirations), and the more dedicated we are to achieving our goals, the less likely we will deviate from social and legal norms. The uncertainty of "getting caught" and losing everything that we have worked for (i.e., employment, education, relationships, etc.) is too great to risk when one's commitment to conventionality is strong. Third, the more a person is *involved* in conventional activity, the less time he/she will have to participate in deviant or criminal activity. Last, if one's *beliefs* strongly adhere to conventional social and legal norms, the less likely one is to violate them. However, once these beliefs become weakened and the person no longer feels he/she must adhere to these rules, the more likely he/she is to break them.

In Hirschi's study of urban male teens in California, the strongest evidence cited for the prevention of delinquent behavior was found among the bonds of attachment, commitment, and belief (Burton, 1991; Hirschi, 1969). In spite of these

---

[1] This is known as contextualism.

findings, many theorists pointed to flaws in his conclusions. Hirschi was criticized for examining minor forms of delinquent behavior (Burton, 1991), for failing to account for background factors (i.e., social class) (Wiatrowski et al., 1981), for assuming that delinquency affects all juveniles the same regardless of differences in age (LaGrange & White, 1985) and for the invariable composition of his sample size (only juveniles and only males were represented) (Burton, 1991). His finding that attachment to delinquent peers does not contribute to higher rates of delinquency was disproved by those who attempted to replicate his study (Burton, 1991; Hindelang, 1973). It appears that not all attachments are beneficial and if a juvenile attaches to delinquent peers, his/her chances of engaging in delinquency increases (see Edwin Sutherland's Theory of Differential Association, 1949).

Other researchers who examined control theory found support for some of Hirschi's variables. The problems for replication, however, were attributed to the means used to operationalize the different bonds. Burton (1991) stated that those who tested control theory only formulated minor modifications to Hirschi's original theory. Researchers may have looked at different samples, different forms of delinquency, or utilized longitudinal data but made no major modifications to its original inception. In his literature review of 22 studies that tested control theory, only two studies did not find any support for the theory (see Agnew, 1985; Torstensson, 1990). The 20 studies that showed support for social control discovered that attachment and belief had the strongest supportive evidence, while involvement was the least supported among the four bonds. When Burton constructed a literature review of researchers that tested two or more theories (including social control), he found nine that supported control theory, 18 that supported differential association or learning theory over social control, and nine that found support for both. Hindelang (1973) also produced findings that were consistent with Hirschi's findings. Attachment to parents, teachers, and schools, a commitment to conventional activities and beliefs, and strong involvement in school activities, all appeared to be related to reduced rates of delinquency. Conversely, he also determined that peer attachment was positively related to delinquent behavior, while poor attachment to parents appeared to be the strongest predictor of delinquency among males. Similarly, Wiatrowski et al. (1981) stated that parental and school attachment, involvement in conventional activities, and maintaining conventional beliefs were all related to decreased delinquent activity. Delinquency was also associated with disorganization and instability in the home (Osborn, 1980).

Many other theorists have found at least partial support for social control theory. Some have discovered that school success is more important than parental attachment (Johnson, 1979), some have maintained that there is no relationship between delinquency and involvement/commitment to conventional activities (Burton, 1991), some have established supportive relationships between reduced rates of delinquency and strong conventional beliefs (Burton, 1991), and others have stated that social control can explain some types of crime, but is poor in explaining other types of criminal activity (Burton, Cullen, Evans, Alarid, & Dunaway, 1998; Rosenbaum, 1987). For example, Rosenbaum stated that social control theory can explain drug use better than it can explain violent crimes or property crimes, whereas

Shover, Norland, James, and Thornton (1979) stated that the bonds of attachment and belief are related to both property offenses and aggressive crimes. Friedman and Rosenbaum (1988) held that weak parental bonds were associated with crimes like robbery and assault, while a weak commitment to school was associated with property offenses. Those with delinquent associates/attachments were more likely to commit both serious and property offenses.

Life course theory emphasizes the quality and strength of social bonds in modifying criminal trajectories. Like Hirschi, life course theorists maintain that weak attachments to family and school can lead to delinquent behavior (Sampson & Laub, 1993). Poor parental supervision and poor parent/child relationships can contribute to early bouts of delinquent activity (McCord, 1986), and conduct disorder problems in childhood have been associated with ineffective child rearing and a subsequent breakdown in the family structure (Farrington, Loeber, & Van Kammen, 1990). Nevertheless, juveniles are not the only ones affected by weak social bonds. Strong social bonds in adulthood can lead to changes in the life course. Sampson and Laub stated,

> Adult social ties are important insofar as they create interdependent systems of obligation and restraint that impose significant costs from translating criminal propensities into action. By contrast, those subjected to weak systems of interdependent and informal social controls as an adult are freer to engage in deviant behavior—even if non delinquent as a youth. This dual premise allows us to explain desistance from crime as well as late onset (p. 141).

Delinquency has a cumulative effect on adult criminal careers, known as "cumulative continuity." Antisocial behavior in childhood and delinquent behavior during adolescence can contribute to adult patterns of offending by severing adult social bonds and further isolating the individual from conventional society (Laub & Sampson, 1993). The longer one engages in delinquency, the more isolated one becomes from conventional society, the less social capital he/she maintains, and the more difficult it is to reestablish conventional connections. In regard to cumulative continuity, individuals can be drawn into situations or environments that bolster their deviant/antisocial personality traits (i.e., associating with criminal peers), which helps to maintain and strengthen them (Caspi & Bem, 1990; Caspi, Elder, & Herbener, 1990; Caspi, Ben, & Elder, 1989).

Research supports life course theory. Sampson and Laub (1993) found that those individuals with low job stability, particularly those between the ages of 17 and 25, were more likely to be arrested than those who possessed high job stability. Moreover, those possessing high aspirations for educational and occupational success, and those who had a strong attachment to their spouse, were less likely to be delinquent. Strong marriages (Gibbens, 1984; Sampson & Laub, 1996; Yeager, 2003a), purposeful employment, strong attachments to family (Sampson & Laub, 1996; Yeager, 2003a, 2003b), and working within the military (Elder, 1986; Sampson & Laub, 1990, 1996) were all found to provide positive turning points in the life course of the criminal offender (Laub & Sampson, 1993). "A change in relationships may produce a turning point, a redirection of the life course" (Elder, 2000, p. 1617). It is not just marriage per se that decreases criminality, it is strong marital bonds that help to decrease crime gradually (Laub, Nagin, & Sampson, 1998). Those who are married and stayed married are the least likely to engage in criminal offending, more likely to become home owners, and less likely to go out nightly and engage in heavy drinking and drugging behaviors (Farrington & West, 1995). Not surprisingly, separation from one's spouse was found to be related to criminal behavior (Farrington & West, 1995).

Social Control, Life Course, and the Female Offender

Female criminality is often been neglected as a source of study for many researchers. Although it has not been completely disregarded, it has not reached the significance that characterizes male criminality (Smith & Paternoster, 1987). Many authors chose to ignore the female offender or generated theories of male criminality/deviance and later tried to transfer those theories to the female offender without empirical evidence. "Female criminality has often ended up as a footnote to works on men that purport to be works on criminality in general" (Klein, 1973, p. 3). Since men have dominated the field of sociology, there are sexist influences on sociological research (Schur, 1984). "Women are no longer invisible, but their presence is infrequently and poorly misrepresented" (Daly, 1995, p. 445).

In the life course literature, female sample size is often too small or the follow-up period is often too short to conduct any worthwhile analyses (Block, Blokland, & Nieuwbeerta, 2007). Theorists have failed to recognize behavioral differences between the sexes. Theories that explain male criminality may not adequately explain the behaviors of their female counterparts. These differences can influence successful preventative and/or rehabilitative treatment modalities for women. Furthermore, preventative efforts or treatment modalities derived from theories based on male behavior will not necessarily address the needs of female clients. Researchers are still unsure if the same factors that contribute to male desistance equally contribute to female desistance. "What is known about recidivism comes almost exclusively from studies of men" (Harm & Phillips, 2001). Some theorists believe that without adequate evidence to support the lack of generalizability of criminological theories to female offenders, the call for "gender-specific" crime theories "is premature" (Smith & Paternoster, 1987, p. 142). Nonetheless, female offenders tend to have different medical and social needs than their male counterparts and appear to have different pathways leading them to crime.

Without adequate explanations of female criminality or deviance, readers and researchers alike have been forced to focus their attention on the works of a few. Rosenbaum (1987) believes that social control theory can help to explain female delinquency better than male delinquency particularly when we consider that young males typically enjoy greater freedoms than young females. He states, "Because a greater expectation to conform is placed on females, they require an extra push to break the law. Thus, for a female to engage in delinquent behavior, her bond to society must be weakened to a greater degree than would be necessary for a male" (pp. 129–130). For Covington (1985), social control also explains female criminality better than male criminality. Lack of parental supervision will have more of an effect on female behavior and "social disorganization seems to have far more causal significance for females than males" (p. 350).

Hagan, Simpson, and Gillis (1979) differentiated between informal and formal methods of social control. According to their work, females are governed by more informal controls than their male counterparts due to the fact that parents, more specifically the mothers, have more of an ability to control their daughters than their sons. Strong family relationships appear particularly important in controlling deviant behavior among adolescent girls (Sepsi, 1974). Attachment to parents was a strong predictor of criminal behavior for both males and females, but it was stronger in preventing violent crimes among women (Alarid, Burton, & Cullen, 2000). The child–parental bond has an effect on both male and female crime trajectories. Children who have a healthy relationship with their parents (i.e., they have strong emotional attachments to their parents and they spend quality time with their parents) are less likely to engage in delinquent behavior when compared to children who have poor relationships with their parents (Worthen, 2011). These two factors (time and attachment) are more important in preventing delinquency (especially for girls) than time spent by parents monitoring behavior; overall, parental supervision appeared less important.

In terms of race, Austin (1978) found that a father's absence from the home had more of a devastating effect on Caucasian girls when compared to their African-American counterparts. However, a mother's affection was found to be significantly related to deviance for both white and black girls, and helped to inhibit deviant behavior regardless of the father's presence in the home. For women offenders overall, their relationships with their children and the rest of their family were an important component in the desistance process (Harm & Phillips, 2001). Concomitantly, other theorists have not found any evidence that social control can better predict female criminality over male criminality (Canter, 1982; Jensen & Eve, 1976).

Since females have lower rates of offending than males in all categories of crime, with the one notable exception of prostitution, many traditionally based criminological theories cannot adequately explain the gender gap between the sexes (Steffensmeier & Allan, 1996). "They also lack sensitivity to the manner in which the criminal behavior of women differs from that of men in terms of paths to crime (e.g., prior experience as victims) and in terms of context" (Steffensmeier & Allan 1996, p. 473). It appears that researchers understand more about the factors that can lead to criminality for women (i.e., being a survivor of domestic violence, early childhood abuse, sexual and racial discrimination in adulthood, etc.), but the desistance process for females still remains a mystery (Katz, 2000).

Information regarding female specific trajectories is sparse. Specific gendered research showed that most women do not follow the life course persistent pathway; unlike males, most fall within the adolescence-limited category (Moffitt, Caspi, Rutter, & Silva, 2001). Desistance differs according to gender; girls desist earlier than boys (Graham & Bowling, 1995). Some studies showed a strong relationship between having children and desistance for female offenders, whereas the same did not hold true for male offenders (Brown & Bloom, 2009; Michalsen, 2011). Children may not always work favorably toward the desistance process considering that child care, particularly upon release, is a cause of considerable stress for female offenders. As a result, female offenders cite other factors in their desistance process such as their wish to maintain their sobriety, their need to avoid the negative experiences associated with future incarcerations, and their reliance upon spirituality (Michalsen, 2011). Level of education and attachment to a partner also affects the desistance process for adult women (Graham & Bowling, 1995).

Work and Desistance

For those who are formerly incarcerated, establishing strong bonds to the workplace can serve as a transition. It begins with the belief that their work allows them to achieve a higher purpose in life and serves as an important life transition to encourage desistance. This would include positions that focus on helping others, particularly those that have been through similar life experiences. In a study distinguishing criminal *desisters* from criminal *persisters*, Maruna (2001) found that in order for ex-offenders to maintain the process of desistance or what he terms "making good," they need to be able to find a higher purpose in life, while subsequently making sense out of their life histories. Many desisters expressed a strong desire to provide assistance and support to other offenders or substance users as a way of "giving back." By helping others, they are able to reform their past, recreate their self-identities, and finally accomplish a certain level of success.

For offenders to desist in criminal behavior, they need to find others who will applaud their new conventional efforts (Sommers, Baskin, & Fagan, 1994). They may want to make a change but if they are unable to achieve a new identity and a new network that supports such an identity, they could revert to preexisting criminal networks that will provide them with approval and a sense of individuality. In a study of female desisters in New York City (1994), Sommers et al. stated, "Overall, the success of identity transformation hinges on the women's abilities to establish and maintain commitments and involvements in conventional aspects of life. As the women began to feel accepted and trusted within some conventional social circles, their determination to exit from crime was strengthened, as were their social and personal identities as noncriminals" (p. 144). These conventional circles may also include strong relationships with one's probation or parole officer, which may help ameliorate some of the stress associated with reintegration, in addition to providing encouragement for conventional behaviors, subsequently decreasing the rate of recidivism (Andrews & Kiessling, 1980).

Working in the field of HIV/AIDS within the prison system and/or upon release allows peers from ACE/CARE to "give back" to others and helps them to establish a higher purpose in life. This notion of "giving back" begins behind the walls for women in ACE/CARE, and for many of them, it will continue outside of the walls, providing them with a sense of purpose upon release. The true rehabilitative effect of this type of vocational programming may not only be attributed to the marketable job skills it can provide offenders, but also to the higher purpose it allows them to obtain.

Conclusion

Life course and social control theories offer many valuable explanations for our question of "why" some offenders persist in their criminal endeavors and why some chronic offenders may desist from criminal behavior as adults. The quality and strength of social bonds serve as a transition that can divert paths and alter the criminal trajectory. However, one question still remains—can these bonds be established to redirect paths while one is still serving one's time in prison, particularly for the female criminal? It appears that prison programming can serve as the means to establish this redirection. From the current study, we will see that HIV prison-based peer programming is one type of rehabilitative prison program that can serve to strengthen bonds for female offenders, while redirecting their criminal trajectories. Females are able to "make good," "give back" and alter their preexisting criminal identities. They also have a strong peer group to encourage and support this change. This process begins during the course of incarceration and continues upon release.

Chapter 3
Female Offenders and the Inmate Subculture

Introduction

Women "prison" differently than men. Adaptations to the prison environment may differ according to gender but both sexes can become *prisonized*; Modes of adaptation have an effect on maladjustment rates. Inmates begin to adhere to the rules of the inmate code (i.e., no snitching, keeping one's cool, minding one's business, etc.) (Sykes & Messinger, 1960) and become entrenched within the inmate subculture, a culture that is in direct opposition to the conventional rules of the prison and society (Clemmer, 1940). The difference in *prisonization* among the genders appears to lie in the way one adopts to the prison subculture and how intently one adheres to the *inmate code*. As a survival mechanism, female inmates tend to recreate family, while male inmates enlist as gang members.

Theories of Prison Adaptation

There are two competing theories on the inmate subculture which help to explain rates of maladjustment among prisoners. First, the *deprivation hypothesis* states that inmates embrace the inmate subculture as a way to cope with the pains of imprisonment (i.e., loss of family, loss of freedom, loss of identity, etc.) created by the oppressive conditions of the prison experience (Clemmer, 1940; Sykes, 1958). Second, the *cultural importation hypothesis* states that inmates bring this culture with them when they enter the prison environment (Heffernan, 1972; Irwin & Cressey, 1962). There is empirical support for both models in the literature (Cao, Zhao, & Van Dine, 1997). However, the importation model appears to have more support than the deprivation hypothesis (McCorkle, Miethe, & Drass, 1995). Others find that the deprivation hypothesis is more applicable to male inmates, while the importation hypothesis is more applicable to female inmates (Bowker, 1981;Pollock-Byrne, 1990). These researchers believe that the importation model explains the

K. Collica, *Female Prisoners, AIDS, and Peer Programs: How Female Offenders Transform Their Lives*, SpringerBriefs in Psychology, DOI 10.1007/978-1-4614-5110-5_3, © The Author 2013

creation of the female "play family" better than the deprivation hypothesis because women bring these roles with them from the community into the prison environment (Pollock-Byrne, 1990).

Prisonization

Both men and women can adopt various roles in the inmate subculture to survive the pains of imprisonment (see Heffernan, 1972; Schrag, 1944; Sykes & Messinger, 1960). This issue of prison adaptation is of great concern for prison administrators. The way one adapts or does not adapt to the prison environment can directly impact the inmate's behavior and lead to increased disciplinary problems. This can create safety issues for both staff and inmate population. The more "prisonized" one becomes, the more difficulty one will have in successfully reintegrating back into society (Clemmer, 1940; Irwin & Cressey, 1962), posing a safety issue for the general public.

Prisonization and disciplinary problems are correlated with numerous factors. Adjustment to prison may vary by the characteristics of a particular individual, the type of prison one is housed in, and the types of friends or acquaintances one associates with during one's incarceration (Goodstein & Wright, 1989). Studies supporting the deprivation hypothesis indicated that the most severe pain and/or deprivation for women in prison is the separation from their children (Jones, 1993; McCarthy, 1980; Pollock-Byrne, 1990).

Play Families

According to one of the earliest studies of the female inmate subculture, Giallombardo (1966) found that women suffered from the deprivation hypothesis and, as a coping mechanism, would re-create family units inside of the prison walls. Giallombardo's study was conducted in 1966, but many of her findings are still applicable today. In a more recent study, Jones (1993) found that females in a Midwestern facility adapted to the prison culture through the creation of "play families," and in a small number of circumstances, same sex coupling existed. These couples, however, appeared to fulfill more emotional than sexual needs. While both males and females suffer from the pain of being denied the ability to engage in heterosexual relationships while in prison, most female to female inmate sexual relationships are consensual and are often established to fulfill emotional needs. On the contrary, homosexual relationships in male prisons are often coercive or due to some sort of exchange and/or arrangement between parties (i.e., sex for protection, for goods, etc.) (Bowker, 1981; Pollock-Byrne, 1990). Most women who engage in same sex relationships in prison will not continue to engage in same relationships after they are released, making this one way women adapt to incarceration (Pollock-Byrne, 1990). Additionally, females do not seem to have the same racial problems that exist in male facilities, and while leadership in male facilities is often tied to gang affiliations, women function in smaller groups, like the "pseudo family" (Pollock-Byrne, 1990).

These families are referred to in the literature as "play families" or "pseudo families"; they are created rather than biologically determined. There can be a *jail-mom* and *jail-dad* with *jail-children*. You can have *jail-siblings, jail-aunts, jail-uncles*, etc. Women feel the pains of imprisonment more harshly than males because of the difficulty in being separated from their family and children. A way to deal with this grief is to try and re-create that lost family in prison. This can include the development of consensual same sex relationships, in which one inmate will portray the father figure, typically known as the *butch* or *aggressor*, and one inmate will portray the mother figure, typically known as the *femme. Jail-parents* can assist their *jail-children* in adapting to the inmate subculture and they may prevent them from engaging in troublesome behaviors, while also teaching them how to navigate the prison environment.

Other recent works since Giallombardo have mixed results regarding play families. "Play families" appear to be unique to female American correctional institutions, with little or no evidence of this existing in other countries (Humphrey, 1987). Although the American prison creation of the "play family" is found in more recent research, the nature of America's prison "play family" may be evolving. Propper (1982) found that same sex marriages among female inmates were rare and that most family units consisted of jail-sisters, or jail-mothers and their jail-daughters. Contrary to prior belief, being in a "make-believe" family did not increase one's chances of engaging in a same sex relationship. She cautions that research into the female inmate subculture needs to discriminate between "make-believe" families and same sex partnerships that are often perceived as family units; both are very different ways of adapting to the prison environment. Research not only shows that many female inmates have stopped recreating the traditional prison families, but many feel that they cannot even develop genuine friendships in a prison environment. A proportion of female inmates today feel that they cannot trust other inmates and that any sort of friendship is simply another form of manipulation (Genders & Player, 1990).

Females have different experiences during their incarceration than their male counterparts. So while both groups can become *prisonized*, the way that they "prison" is very different. The pains of imprisonment for women can include disparities in disciplinary practices (women receive more tickets than men for minor infractions), inadequate health care, insufficient therapeutic services (particularly in lieu of the high rates of physical, mental, and sexual abuse among this population), limited educational/vocational programming, risk of sexual abuse by correctional staff, and pains associated with the separation from their children (Owen, 2004).

Both male and female inmates suffer from the pain of being separated from their families, but the separation is more detrimental for women. Even if female inmates are able to have contact with their biological family while incarcerated, their visits, their phone calls, and their mail are closely monitored (Genders & Player, 1990), not allowing for any of the pains of imprisonment (i.e., separation from one's family) to be ameliorated. Since the number of female facilities is significantly smaller than the number of male facilities (many states only have one female facility), women experience additional deprivations because of the inability to transfer to another prison for programmatic needs, problems in the facility (either with staff or with other inmates), or for family matters (MacKenzie, Robinson, & Campbell, 1989). Moreover, most state facilities are located in rural areas, far away from urban cities, where most of the inmates' family live, making a closer to home transfer impossible, thereby increasing the pains of separation from their biological family units.

With prison being so far away from the inmate's family, family contact is severely limited because of the costs in time and money in traveling up to the prison (Reed & Reed, 2004). Collect phone calls are an additional expense and although many families may want to hear from their incarcerated loved ones, they cannot afford to do so. When males are incarcerated, it is typically the women who will bring the children to the facility to see the father, but when most women are incarcerated, another female member of her family will take responsibility for her children. The additional costs of raising this woman's children make amenities like visits, phone calls, and packages extremely limited.

According to the Bureau of Justice Statistics (Snell & Morton, 1994), it is estimated that approximately 1.5 million children in the USA have a parent who is incarcerated. Seventy-five percent of women in prison have children, with almost 70% having a child under the age of 18. This report stated that 25% of the women in prison have children who are living with their biological father, while 90% of the men stated that their children were living with the biological mother. This illustrates that incarcerating mothers has more of an effect on children, resulting in multiple placements, than the subsequent incarceration of fathers.

Subculture Membership

Subculture membership is not static. The subculture that inmates join during their incarceration can be rejected shortly before one's release, changing their investment in such friendships or groups (Wheeler, 1961). In a study of 121 female inmates, Larson and Nelson (1984) found that friendships changed during the course of incarceration and became less important when a woman was near her release date. Greer (2000) discovered similar findings in a study of Midwestern female inmates. Although many female inmates engaged in sexual relationships with other female inmates, there was a great amount of distrust between them. Most of these relationships began, and continued, on the basis of economic motives or loneliness. Distrust existed among nonsexual relationships as well, with most of the women believing that their prison friendships were superficial and would not last outside of the prison environment.

Emotional Responsiveness

Women as a whole, incarcerated or free, appear to be more closely connected with the people around them than their male counterparts. Although men may know more people than women know, women appear to be more aware of problems with their friends and family, and more influenced by such problems, making them more "emotionally responsive" than men (Kessler & McLeod, 1984, p. 628). These emotional responses can be detrimental inside of the prison, since such outbursts are likely to be perceived as a disciplinary problem.

In general, correctional staff believe that female inmates possess a different emotional makeup than male inmates (McClellan, 1994). In a study of NYS (New York State) correctional workers (Pollock, 1984), correctional staff stated that female inmates were more emotional than male inmates, whether they were expressing good or bad emotions. These expressions of emotions were perceived as emotional outbursts that could lead to a ticket (inmates are given tickets for violating prison rules) for verbal assault on an officer. What may be perceived as a normal expression of emotion by the inmate is now perceived as a disciplinary infraction by correctional staff. Staff believed that they had to be more sensitive in dealing with female inmates to avoid such outbursts. They felt that this same type of sensitivity was not necessary in dealing with the male inmate. There is an "assumption that women are irrational, compulsive and slightly neurotic" (Smart, 1976), in addition to being "too emotional," "too manipulative," and "too vocal" (DeBell, 2001, p. 59). Women appeared to be more expressive and more communicative, while men appeared to be more closed and less verbal (Cranford & Williams, 1998).

Women inmates are more expressive about their anger than male inmates (Suter, Byrne, Byrne, Howells, & Day, 2002). These expressions, although nonviolent in nature, may be perceived by staff as constituting a disciplinary infraction, such as insubordination, creating a disturbance, verbal harassment of an officer, or even inciting a riot. Since men and women express themselves differently, what may actually be a healthy way of releasing pent up emotions may be perceived as problematic behavior for the female inmate. Therefore, staff training should focus on communicating effectively with female offenders to avoid unnecessary disciplinary action (DeBell).

Prison Adaptation and Misconduct

The way one adapts to the subculture can have a significant impact on one's disciplinary record, even though there may be better ways of dealing with problematic behaviors other than writing inmates up for infractions (Toch & Grant, 1989). Writing an inmate for an infraction tells the inmate that his/her behavior was unacceptable, but it does not help him/her to correct or modify that behavior. There are many factors associated with high rates of maladjustment, and subsequently high rates of disciplinary infractions. In a study of 883 Ohio-based inmates, Cao et al. (1997) found more support for the importation model over the deprivation hypothesis in explaining the rate of disciplinary infractions. The behaviors that inmates brought into the prison environment appeared to be related to increased misconduct, rather than the oppressive conditions of the prison being blamed for begetting such misconduct. There appears to be more violations in the first year of prison, with the rate of violations decreasing after the first year, but the seriousness of violations increasing after the first year (Lindquist, 1980).

Age

Age appears to be a factor that is significantly correlated with the rate of infractions. Wolfgang (1961) found that those over the age of 35 were more adjusted to prison than those under the age of 35. As one increases in age, one will decrease in problematic behavior and decrease in the severity of infractions (Jensen, 1977; Jensen & Jones, 1976; MacKenzie, 1987; Wolf, Freinek, & Shaffer, 1966). It was also found that at a certain point (age 27), the rate of infractions will begin to increase once more, negating the inverse relationship between age and rate of disciplinary infractions.

Race

The relationship between race and rate of infractions is not fully understood. Inmates of color, both male and female, are more likely to receive disciplinary infractions than their white counterparts (Cao et al., 1997; Lindquist, 1980; Poole & Regoli, 1980), although this finding is inconsistent (Hewitt, Poole, & Regoli, 1984; Stephan, 1989). Casey-Acevedo and Bakken (2003) found that African–American female inmates were more likely to receive a disciplinary infraction for violent misconduct (i.e., assault) than Caucasian women. Race may affect who receives an infraction but it does not appear to affect the severity of punishment received (Ramirez, 1983).

Sentence Length

Sentence length has been another factor associated with the rate of disciplinary infractions, illustrating that long-termers are involved in less infractions than short-termers (Flanagan, 1980). Others have found that those with shorter sentences appear to have an easier adjustment than those with longer sentences (MacKenzie & Goodstein, 1985). There appears to be more violations in the first year of prison, with the rate of violations decreasing after the first year, but the seriousness of violations increasing after the first year (Lindquist, 1980). Those with longer sentences experience more stress and more difficulty in adjustment at the beginning of their sentence than those long-termers who have already served a significant portion of their time (MacKenzie & Goodstein, 1995). Some researchers have not found a difference in stress levels between long term and short term offenders, with both groups perceiving similar issues and problems (Richards, 1978) and experiencing the same modes of adjustment (Wolfgang, 1961). While Wheeler (1961) found a correlation between sentence length and prisonization, Atchley and McCabe (1968) found that conformity to prison rules was higher after 6 months of incarceration. The authors state that the differences in results may be due to the study of different inmate populations (i.e., state vs. federal inmates).

In a study of female offenders in Louisiana (MacKenzie et al., 1989), women with shorter sentences often had fears of personal safety, while those with longer sentences were more likely to engage in "play families." Concomitantly, there was a connection between adjustment and prior incarcerations and adjustment and marriage. Those who have never been married and those who have never been to prison before were more likely to have adjustment problems when compared to those inmates who were married and served prior prisons sentences (Wolfgang, 1961). For women offenders, short-termers and long-termers have similar psychological makeups (Long et al., 1984), yet, still engage in varying patterns of rule breaking behavior. For female offenders, short-termers (serving less than 18 months) commit mostly minor infractions which tend to increase during incarceration, while long-termers, both minor and serious rule breakers, engage in most of their misconduct during the early part of their sentence, with rates of misconduct decreasing as time in prison increases (Casey-Acevedo, 2001).

Inmate Perception, Mental Illness & Intelligence

How the inmates perceive their environment may affect disciplinary behavior. The less control they feel that they have over their environment, the more maladjusted they appear to be (Wright, 1999). If they are involved in programs and other activities, and feel that their safety is not in jeopardy, the less stress they will experience and the less likely they will engage in problematic behaviors (Wright, 1999). The presence of a mental illness can complicate such matters. Those with a mental illness tend to violate more prison rules, and the greater the illness, the greater the number of violations (Toch & Adams, 1986). An inmate's mental illness can hinder his/her ability to adhere to prison rules. However, many inmates, if left undiagnosed, will be punished for violating such rules. Their misconduct is a manifestation of their mental illness but perceived by staff as a blatant disregard for rules and authority. Mental illness is not related to one's level of intelligence. Nevertheless, there is no relationship between one's intelligence level and one's rate of institutional misconduct (Wolf et al., 1966).

Disciplinary Infractions

In a report compiled by the Bureau of Justice Statistics (Stephan, 1989), over half of all inmates were found guilty of violating prison rules. The average rate of inmate infractions was 1.5 per year. Those who were younger, incarcerated in larger institutions or maximum security institutions, unmarried, serving time for a property offense or a robbery, having a past history of incarceration, having been arrested for the first time as a juvenile, having less than a high school diploma or GED, and having a history of drug misuse were more likely to receive infractions than other types of inmates. Others found that age at commitment, drug use history, and serving time for a homicide were related to varying rates of misconduct among inmates (Flanagan, 1983). In comparing disciplinary infractions across institutions, Brown and Spevacek (1971) found that correctional officers in different facilities write approximately the same number of tickets but the reasons for writing them may differ by institution.

Research showed that female inmates were more likely to receive disciplinary infractions than male inmates (Cao et al., 1997; Stephan, 1989), even though the levels of violence in female institutions are significantly lower than levels of violence in male institutions (Kruttschnitt & Krmpotich, 1990; Lindquist, 1980). Women commit less serious violations than men, even though they are cited for infractions regularly (Casey-Acevedo & Bakken, 2003). Female inmates are often written up for minor infractions. Both male and female inmates are cited most often for disobeying a direct order (Tischler & Marquart, 1989). It is estimated, though, that females are twice as likely as males to be written up for such minor infractions (Eaton, 1993). Women incurred approximately 2 infractions per year, while their male counterparts incurred 1.4 per year (Stephan, 1989). Behavior that is often ignored in male facilities is severely enforced and punished in female institutions (Dobash, Dobash, & Gutteridge, 1986). In a study of Texas female inmates conducted by McClellan (1994), the most frequent infraction for male and female inmates was insubordination. The women in this study, however, received written reprimands, which is a form of discipline only found in female institutions, subjecting them to an additional form of institutional control and punishment. She found that while 87% of the women in her sample received written reprimands, none of the men received any written reprimands. Although women committed less serious infractions, they were punished more severely than the male inmates. This higher form of scrutiny will lead to a higher number of overall infractions for the female offender, which will affect her ability to obtain early release.

Leger (1987) found that gay women were more likely to receive disciplinary infractions than straight women and they were more likely to follow the inmate code. The inmate aggressor may be penalized more often for perceived problematic behaviors because she comes to the attention of correctional staff more easily. Inadvertently, she could be penalized for continuously violating gender norms, which may be viewed as a threat to correctional staff, consisting mostly of male workers. Generally, it is really difficult to know the true rate of infractions among inmates, considering that the writing of an infraction is based entirely upon the discretion of the correctional officer or civilian staff member (Casey-Acevedo & Bakken, 2003). Inmates commit more infractions than recorded by official data and it appears that correctional officers do not officially report a majority of the infractions (Hewitt et al., 1984). Correctional officers decide which behavior constitutes a rule infraction and which inmate will be punished for which behavior (Poole & Regoli, 1980). Therefore, it is quite plausible that younger inmates, inmates of color, those serving shorter sentences, etc. are not committing more infractions than other types of inmates. It could simply be that these inmates are more visible to correctional staff, thereby receiving a higher level of scrutiny, and having a higher chance of getting caught and punished for such behavior. This specifically applies to female offenders, where their behavior is no worse than that of their male counterparts, but their behavior comes to the attention of correctional staff more easily. "When staff expect women to be more troublesome than men, and expand more energy in the detection and punishment of their misbehaviors, it is little wonder that women have high disciplinary rates" (Humphrey, 1987, p. 5).

Prison Adaptation Through ACE and CARE

ACE and CARE can provide female offenders with conventional identities and motivate them to engage in a different, more conventional form of adaptation, which inadvertently aids in rebuking the inmate code. In addition to finding a higher purpose and possessing the desire to change, for successful desistance to occur, female offenders need to find others who will applaud their new conventional efforts (Sommers, Baskin, & Fagan, 1994). In an environment that can often be hostile and filled with humiliating procedures (i.e., strip searches, verbal abuse, violence, etc.), inmates are exposed to many negative influences behind bars that can negate the rehabilitative effects that prison is supposed to employ (LPSSC, 2004). Offenders may want to make a change, but if they are unable to achieve a new identity and a new network that supports such an identity, they could revert to preexisting criminal networks that will provide them with approval, a sense of self worth, and a sense of familiarity. It is a widely shared belief that when people go to prison they can learn to become better criminals (Sommers et al., 1994). However, even in the midst of the prison environment, it is possible to establish strong relationships with conventional others and these relationships do not have to be based on superficiality.

Programs for female offenders can assist in providing inmates with strong conventional support from one another during incarceration (Koons, Burrow, Morash, & Bynum, 1997). For the women working in ACE and CARE, these conventional relationships can be formed and maintained by the ACE/CARE civilian staff and the peer workers during the course of incarceration, but it is only supposed to be continued after release by the ACE/CARE civilian staff. If the women are caught maintaining relationships with the other ACE/CARE peers after leaving prison, who are women who would applaud and encourage their efforts on the outside just as they did on the inside, they run the risk of committing a parole violation by "associating with another known felon." This rule, which is mandated by the Division of Parole, was obviously set forth to reduce the chance of inmates connecting with one another on the outside to commit crime. However, if the women form conventional relationships on the inside with other offenders, and these relationships must be severed upon release, we run the risk of promoting criminal behavior; they are forced to ignore those who would unwittingly support their new conventional identities.

Research indicated that strong social networks and a high level of "social capital" are essential for successful reintegration for female offenders (Reisig, Holtfreter, & Morash, 2002). This proves to be even more vital for younger offenders and those offenders with few financial resources, considering they have been found to have lower levels of social support, thereby increasing their chance for recidivism

(Reisig et al. 2002). For many of the women in ACE/CARE, this may be the only positive social network that they have ever developed. Without it, their chances of success appear to dwindle and their new self-identity may be lost.

Prior research supported the notion that releasees feel more comfortable receiving support from others who were formerly incarcerated. In a study of female prisons in England and Wales, Eaton (1993) found that many women enjoyed being involved with organizations after release that would employ ex-offenders because it gave them "a sense of belonging" (p. 66). Working in programs like ACE/CARE allows the peers to form conventional relationships and attachments, and it helps to prevent one from becoming "institutionalized" or "prisonized," which can hamper rates of institutional and post-release success. The process of "prisionization" or "institutionalization" can beget maladjustment problems, hence increasing disciplinary infractions during incarceration and decreasing levels of success upon release. It is evident that another rehabilitative effect of this type of vocational programming may not only be attributed to the marketable job skills it can provide offenders and the higher purpose it allows them to obtain, but in its ability to lessen the effects of "prisonization." By cultivating strong conventional attachments and strong networks of support, which begin behind the walls but continue outside of them, the women of ACE/CARE can easily adopt the role of the "wounded healer" or "professional ex" and be supported, unconditionally, in their new conventional role.

Conclusion

Programs such as ACE and CARE may provide a conventional inmate culture and conventional code for female offenders to follow. If ACE/CARE serves as an extended family unit for female inmates, it can help ameliorate some of the pains of imprisonment but it can do so in a positive manner. These women may find the family that they are seeking in a supportive and nurturing environment, which will not only help to give them a higher purpose in life, but also provide accolades for the establishment of their newfound conventional identity. Since one's associates in prison can affect adjustment, being associated with programs like ACE/CARE can prevent periods of maladjustment at the beginning and end of one's sentence, where disciplinary infractions appear to be their highest. The women in these programs provide leadership, support, and guidance for one another, and if the women are viewed as role models by other inmates and correctional staff, they are less likely to jeopardize their position by engaging in unlawful or deviant behaviors. A study conducted by Fox (1984) at Bedford Hills Correctional Facility found that the decrease in "play families" was correlated with an increase in vocational and educational programming. If prison administrators and researchers are concerned about the problems associated with prisonization, providing inmates with purposeful employment while incarcerated may combat this issue.

Chapter 4
The Effects of Prison-Based Programming

Introduction

Rehabilitation advocates argue that prison programs teach valuable skills and these skills are necessary if prisoners have any chance of leading productive lives after prison. Retributivists argue that educational services do not lead to rehabilitative goals; hence, they should be abolished or restricted. Despite the current trend toward retribution, we are ignoring studies that show that educational/vocational programming can have significant positive effects for the inmate and for the community in which he/she will reside in after release. Our goal should not simply be to "warehouse" offenders if there is evidence that rehabilitative goals are possible. Our goal should be to enhance prison programming because there is an abundance of evidence that links these programs to positive post-release outcomes. These positive outcomes will benefit everyone economically and socially. It is clear from the research that prison programming can serve as a life course transition and possibly change the criminal trajectory. It is also clear from the current study that one program that has been overlooked as a vocational opportunity to promote criminal desistance is HIV prison-based peer programming.

The History of Prison-Based Programming

Education and rehabilitation was integral to the reformatory's original design. For over 150 years, prison programs were an essential component of the American prison system (Gaes, Flanagan, Motiuk, & Stewart, 1999). Prison programs of the nineteenth century reformatory concentrated on religious teachings and spirituality (Gerber & Fritsch, 1995). Offenders could be rehabilitated and redeemed through God. Illiteracy precluded many offenders from reading and comprehending the teachings of the Bible. The cultivation of academic programs resulted from a need to help offenders read the Bible and understand vital religious materials (Linden &

K. Collica, *Female Prisoners, AIDS, and Peer Programs: How Female Offenders Transform Their Lives*, SpringerBriefs in Psychology, DOI 10.1007/978-1-4614-5110-5_4, © The Author 2013

Perry, 1982). To facilitate religious education, literacy programming in prison was a necessity. Superintendent Zebulon Brockway of the Elmira Reformatory in New York State mandated academic programs for all of his inmates in the late 1800s (Linden & Perry, 1982) but most facilities did not develop their own educational/vocational programming until the 1930s (Gaes et al., 1999; Gerber & Fritsch 1995). A study of correctional facilities from 1927 to 1928 [presented in MacCormick's (1931) report] demonstrated that education was the best tool in the rehabilitation of the criminal (Hunsinger, 1997; MacCormick, 1931).

Educational programming for inmates was commonplace by the 1930s (Linden & Perry, 1982), and in 1945 (after World War II) some prisons started to offer post-secondary education (McCollum, 1994). The 1950s and the 1960s were also very supportive of rehabilitation and prison-based education (Linden & Perry, 1982), with more facilities offering college programming during this time period as a way to lower recidivism (Gaes et al., 1999; Gerber & Fritsch, 1995; Knepper, 1990; Linden & Perry, 1982). Facilities that did not offer secondary education could not afford its costs (Taylor, 1993). By the 1960s, the BEOG (Basic Educational Opportunity Grant), which gave tuition assistance to low income families, was born (Knepper, 1990; McCollum, 1984). This program was later extended to middle-class families and renamed the Pell Grant (McCollum, 1984) when Congress passed Title V of the Higher Education Act in 1965 (Taylor, 1993). Inmates, most of whom were economically disadvantaged prior to incarceration, qualified for this tuition assistance. With financial support from both state and federal governments, college programs burgeoned in American prisons (Ryan & McCabe, 1994). By 1973, there were 182 college programs; these programs grew to 273 by 1976 and, finally, 350 by 1982 (Taylor, 1993). Approximately 90% of states were offering some type of prison-based college programming (Taylor, 1993).

A Return to Retributive Policies

Support for inmate education changed with Martinson's famous 1974 study on the rehabilitative effects of prison-based programming (Lipton, Martinson, & Wilks, 1975). Martinson stated, "With few and isolated exceptions, the rehabilitative efforts that have been reported so far have had no appreciable effect on recidivism, (1974, p. 25)," even though 48% of the programs surveyed indicated rehabilitative outcomes. Martinson stated that prison interventions were fruitless and previous studies that claimed to show a correlation between rehabilitation and recidivism were empirically weak and methodologically unsound. Martinson's study was synonymous with the phrase "nothing works" (Welch, 1996), but in fact, Martinson never used these exact words in his report (Farabee, 2002). Interestingly, in 1979, Martinson changed his original opinion on rehabilitation, but, by this time, prison officials began to doubt the effectiveness of educational and vocational programming in transforming the offender (Knepper, 1990). They used Martinson's original study as evidence of its failure. Martinson was strongly criticized by reformers for coming to these conclusions too quickly. Although his findings lacked empirical support, his claims were regrettably "accepted [as] criminological truth" (Cullen & Gendreau, 1989).

By the 1980s, we witnessed a return to retributive priorities and a sharp reduction in educational funding for prisons (Ryan & McCabe, 1994). Several bills to eliminate all prisoner financial aid were introduced by Republicans. These bills originally failed to gain enough congressional support until former democratic President Bill Clinton signed the Omnibus Crime Bill into law in 1994; the attached rider abolished Pell grants for prisoners (Lewis, 1994; Linton, 1998; Yarbo, 1996). Some programs managed to survive on state financial aid (i.e., TAP—Tuition Assistance Program) but many states followed the federal government's lead and eradicated this source of funding as well (Audeh, 1995). Even before Clinton signed this law into effect, many states already started to restrict funding for postsecondary education. In the 5 years before Pell Grants were eliminated, almost one-half of the states cut educational, vocational, and technological programming budgets (Currie, 1998; Lillis, 1994).

Providing inmates with financial assistance does not take assistance away from those in the community. From 1991 to 1992, less than 0.8% of 1% of all Pell Grants were given to inmates (Taylor, 1992). If all the money saved was evenly divided between all Pell Grant recipients, it would work out to less than five dollars per person per semester (Taylor, 1993). College education is highly cost effective. On average it costs $31,000 to incarcerate one inmate per year (Henrichson & Delaney, 2012) but it only costs $2,500 to provide an inmate with a college degree (Taylor, 1993). When recidivism is reduced, we save taxpayers a substantial amount of money.

For the few prison-based college programs that managed to survive, the budget cuts resulted in longer waiting lists for all programs, larger class sizes, and less course offerings (Lillis, 1994). The remaining college programs tried to defer tuition costs by requiring inmates to pay partial or total tuition fees, either through their personal accounts or through private grants and/or scholarships (Lawrence, Meors, Dubin, & Travis, 2002). Consequently, the number of inmates enrolled in postsecondary programming abruptly diminished. Between 1994 and 1995, "the number of state prison inmates enrolled in post-secondary education dropped from 38,000 to 21,000—this in a population of close to one million. By the 1994–1995 academic year, about half of state prison systems offered some kind of baccalaureate program; by the following year, only a third did" (Currie, 1998, p. 169). Between 1991 and 1997, inmate participation in academic studies decreased from 42% to 35%, and inmate participation in vocational studies decreased from 31% to 27% (Lawrence et al., 2002). Funding provided for special educational services decreased as well, and by 1998, most states eliminated all programmatic prison funding (Correctional Educational Bulletin, 2002).

Politicians focused their energies on reinstating retribution as our correction system's primary goal (i.e., elimination of prison programming, the implementation of three strikes legislation and mandatory minimum sentences, truth in sentencing policies that require inmates to complete at least 85% of their sentence, limiting or suspending parole eligibility or good-time credits, the elimination of parole by many states and the federal system, the move from indeterminate to determinate sentencing, and the return of the chain gang and the black and white stripped uniform) and they used atypical crime stories to induce public panic to support Draconian crime legislation (i.e., the Polly Klass case[1]). Public opinion is often a reaction to politicians highlighting such issues as major social problems (Beckett, 1997). In spite of misinformation, the public is surprisingly supportive of rehabilitation, even if it is secondary to retribution (Applegate, Cullen, & Fisher's, 1997) "...Policy makers consistently overestimate public punitiveness and consistently underestimate public support for rehabilitation" (Applegate et al., p. 250).

The Need for Rehabilitative Programming in Prison

Academic/vocational programs are necessary for prisoners; inmates face far greater deficits than people who reside in the general population. Inmates lack academic skills and illiteracy is commonplace. Nearly one-half of prisoners have below a sixth grade reading level (Tewksbury, 1994), and approximately 75% are virtually illiterate (Tewksbury, 1994; Trites & Fiedorowicz, 1991), compared to a 20% illiteracy rate among the general population (Trites & Fiedorowicz, 1991). One-half of inmates possess a high school diploma (Lawrence et al., 2002; Smith & Silverman 1994; Tewksbury & Vito, 1994), compared to three-fourths of the general population (Lawrence et al., 2002). Inmates tend to trail approximately 2–3 grades behind those who have achieved the same level of formal education (Tewksbury, 1994; Tewksbury & Vito, 1994). The Bureau of Justice Statistics estimates that 40% of state inmates, 27% of federal inmates, and 47% of jail inmates did not possess a high school diploma or GED; in the general population, only 18% of people have not obtained their high school diploma or GED (Harlow, 2003). The IQ levels of offenders are one standard deviation below the nation's average, with slightly less than half (42%) diagnosed with some type of learning disability (Bell, Conard & Suppa, 1984).

In addition to their poor academic skills, prisoners also possess very poor employment skills. Their work history and work skills are far below the national average (Lawrence et al., 2002). When these deficits are combined with the stigma of being an "ex-con," future prospects of long-term employment appear rather bleak (Lawrence et al., 2002). Illiteracy tends to lead to limited opportunities, low self-esteem, frustration, and disorderly behavior (Trites & Fiedorowicz, 1991). Low educational levels do not cause crime but it is definitely a contributing factor (Linton, 1998).

---

[1] Polly Klass was abducted from her bedroom by Richard Allen Davis, a repeat offender. This case fueled the passage of California's Three Strikes Legislation. Stranger abduction of a child is rare but this case was highlighted and used to pass the three strikes legislation, which has not proven to reduce crime rates, but has managed to bankrupt the State of California with the overcrowding of its jails/prisons.

Research on Prison-Based Programming

Numerous studies show that prison-based programming reduces recidivism. All studies, whether they demonstrate a positive or negative correlation between prison-based programming and recidivism, suffer from methodological flaws. Researchers studying prison programs need to consider that inmates are affected by a multitude of factors; we cannot place the onus of responsibility on one program or on one treatment in particular (Lawrence et al., 2002). A combination of different programs may contribute to the inmate's success. Prison-based research often contains small samples, which makes it difficult to generalize findings to others in the same population (Gerber & Fritsch, 1995). Moreover, the way in which program outcomes are measured can be problematic. There are no universally accepted criteria for program assessment. Recidivism is commonly used as an outcome variable but operationalizing this variable effectively is often difficult since there is no universally accepted definition of recidivism (Taylor, 1992).

"Despite methodological shortcomings and challenges, the evidence suggests that carefully designed and administered education and work programs can improve inmates' institutional behavior, reduce recidivism, and promote involvement in prosocial activities after release" (Gaes et al., 1999, p. 398). Since Martinson, there are few studies that show a negative relationship between education and recidivism (Gerber & Fritsch, 1995) but there are necessary components that will make some programs more successful than others. This is attributable to several factors. Successful programs will (1) be separate from the rest of the facility (this minimizes distractions); (2) provide follow-up services (like job placement); and (3) provide skills that are highly marketable in today's job market (Gerber & Fritsch, 1995). In a literature review on prison education, Linden and Perry (1982) found that programs will be most successful if they are "intensive," if they can establish an "alternative community within the prison," and "if they offer post-release services to inmates" (p. 55). Prison-based HIV programs have been able to successfully accomplish all three tasks.

Research indicates that educational level is positively correlated with successful reintegration (Correctional Educational Bulletin, 2002) and reduced recidivism (Shrum, 2004). A plethora of research connects education with positive post-release outcomes (McCollum, 1994). These studies tend to be "methodologically weak but consistently show positive consequences for society" (Gerber & Fritsch, 1995, p. 129). Absent an education, releasees will most likely hold menial jobs with little pay, seek public assistance, or resort back to criminal activity (O'Neil, 1990). Prison-based programming provides inmates a real chance at achieving the conventional American dream (Taylor, 1992).

Education programs are the best way for inmates to learn new skills or to enhance skills they may already have (Tootoonchi, 1993). Studies showed that inmates who participated in college programming were able to obtain higher levels of employment than other releasees, suggesting that education can ameliorate the effects of the ex-offender stigma (Taylor, 1993). Post-secondary correctional education (PSCE) was shown to be effective and efficient (Taylor, 1992).

College graduates had a much greater chance of obtaining stable employment than college dropouts or high school/GED recipients (Taylor, 1992) and they recidivated at a considerably lower rate than inmates who did not earn a degree while incarcerated (Clark, 1991). Even inmates who only possessed a GED fared better after release than those released from prison with less than a GED (Nuttall, Hollmen, & Staley, 2003), particularly if they were under the age of 21 (Staley, 2001). All of these factors are likely to lead to reduced recidivism by increasing literacy, which will lead to increased employment prospects, and "by facilitating the maturation, conscientiousness, and dedication that educational achievement requires" (Gaes et al., 1999, p. 399). "It is no surprise that educational deficiencies are strongly related to criminal activity" (Tewksbury, 1994, p. 398), and studies show a relationship between "underemployment, a career criminal lifestyle, and low academic skills" (Tewksbury, 1994, p. 399).

Improving educational standards for inmates cannot be the only goal of corrections officials. Limited vocational skills are a major hindrance to offender reintegration. "...If an offender possesses a marketable job skill, employer objection to his criminal record is reduced significantly" (Enocksson, 1981, p. 11). Jobs held within the prison system (i.e., porter) have little utility in the outside job market (Schumacker, Anderson, & Anderson, 1990), but vocational training can provide skills that are marketable in today's workforce. Without such training, prisons "run the risk of creating workers whose skills are suited solely to an institutional setting" (Koski, 1998, p. 158). There is strong empirical support between vocational program participation and reduced recidivism (Brandon, 1998; Canestrini, 1993; MacDonald, 1995).

Prison-based programs provide an essential opportunity to open the lines of communication between inmates and positive civilian staff members who help to reinforce law-abiding norms and values (Gaes et al., 1999; Harer, 1995; Taylor, 1992). Staff play a fundamental role in the overall success of a program. Staff characteristics, such as personality and dedication, and the interactions between staff and inmates, can be the difference between a successful program and an unsuccessful program (Koons, Burrow, Morash, & Bynum, 1997; Palmer, 1995). Both the civilians and inmates who participate in these programs serve as positive role models (Taylor, 1992, 1993). Regardless of program type, the staff who provides such programming appears to be the most important factor in an inmate's success. Great success can be obtained with "innovative" programming and "talented" staff (Linden & Perry, 1982). Those who have experience working with this population, and who are familiar with prison/jail policies and procedures, will prove to be the most effective educators (Tewksbury, 1994). Overall, successful programs will have clear objectives and attainable goals (Tewksbury, 1993).

Programs not only affect post-release outcomes; we witness the benefits while offenders are serving their sentences. Educational programs are correlated with a decrease in disciplinary behavior (Taylor, 1993). These programs monopolize the inmates' time and serve to restrict the negative persuasions of prison life (Harer, 1995). Programs provide an incentive for inmates to stay out of trouble (Taylor, 1993), particularly if disciplinary action can lead to the removal from a desired program. Prison programming not only provides a hiatus from the mundane daily routine of prison life (Taylor, 1993) but also helps to raise levels of self-esteem (Tewksbury & Vito, 1994). Self-esteem is an important factor in maintaining a law-abiding life style and it is an important part of rehabilitation and reintegration (Tewksbury & Vito, 1994).

Challenges to Prison-Based Programming

Programs face many challenges within the correctional setting and the ability to overcome these challenges may impact the effectiveness of overall programming. The types of programming offered and the quality of these programs have largely been affected by budgetary constraints and the lack of scientific study (Lawrence et al., 2002). Many programs have been based on "intuition, benevolent intentions, and experience," rather than evidence based (Gaes et al., 1999, p. 399). Programs have to learn to effectively deal with high staff turnover rates, lack of funding, limited space, and learning to accept that they are probably the lowest priority of prison officials (Lawrence et al., 2002). Security overrides all other functions in the prison system and educators need to acclimate to providing services in a rigid environment. Program staff must remain active in recruiting inmates, maintaining inmate involvement in the program, making themselves accessible and known to inmate population, deciding which staff persons are in charge of which responsibilities and adjusting to a jail/prison schedule (Tewksbury, 1994). Programs within the facility should be widely publicized and easily accessible to interested inmates (Schumacker et al., 1990). Even though most prisons and jails offer GED and ABE (Adult Basic Education) programming, the waiting lists are astronomical. There is also a lack of standardization in prison school programs (Schumacker et al., 1990). An inmate may be close to completing an academic degree when he/she is transferred to another facility. The new facility may not offer the same programming, or if they do, the inmate will return to the bottom of the waiting list once again.

Programs may have difficulty establishing efficacious working relationships between all contributing agencies, including the Department of Corrections. These agency partners should agree on a set of program objectives, before program implementation, to prevent confusion or conflict in the future. Unfortunately, the goals of educators and the goals of prison officials appear to be in opposition with each other. The Department of Corrections wishes to maintain "custody and control" while the goals of educators focus on "freedom, growth and self-actualization" (O'Neil, 1990, p. 28). In order for programs to be effective, all parties involved have to make some compromises.

Women Offenders and Prison-Based Programming

The majority of studies conducted on the effectiveness of prison-based programming focus on male inmates. Fortuitously, the few studies that examined females showed the same promising results for men and women after prison-program participation

(Correctional Educational Bulletin, 2001, 2002). In comparing male and female inmates, the greatest disparities exist for vocational opportunities. According to Lahm (2000), male offenders are sent to different facilities based on their security level, their needs, and the programming provided. Most states, however, only have one female facility, limiting the types of program services offered. Many vocational programs for female offenders are gender based and prepare them to work in traditional pink-collar employment for little pay (i.e., secretarial, sewing, food service, etc.). Male offenders are typically trained in traditional blue-collar jobs (air conditioning repair, plumbing, electronics, etc.). Consequently, men are able to obtain better skills, skills that will allow them to obtain better employment opportunities, with higher wages, upon release.

Lahm (2000) examined correctional programming in 30 states (417 male correctional facilities and 47 female correctional facilities) and found that all offered general education programs. This means that basic educational opportunities for women have increased over the last 30 years. Unfortunately, secondary education was on the decline for both men and women; only one-half of the correctional facilities studied offered college courses. In terms of vocational education, more female facilities were offering vocations in professional studies than in the past, but approximately 85% still offered gender-stereotyped programming. Females are still being trained for "unstable" and "underpaid" jobs.

The subservient role of women in society is reflected within the prison environment, as prison is often a larger reflection of societal problems like racism, classism, and sexism. Since women are not afforded as many vocational and educational opportunities as male offenders while in prison, these acquiescent roles are perpetuated by the correctional system in its failure to provide skills equality (Moyer, 1984; Smart, 1976). Due to their smaller numbers, correctional officials have often been able to rationalize circumventing the programmatic needs of female inmates (Bonta, Pang, & Wallace-Capretta, 1995). Even today, most of the jobs that women are assigned to in the prison system focus on domestic work and do not teach the women relevant job skills, but only help in the daily maintenance of the institution (Dobash, Dobash & Gutteridge, 1986; Pollock-Byrne, 1990). This provides no opportunity for rehabilitation or for the attainment of valuable job skills which would afford them the opportunity to be able to support themselves and their family upon release (Pollock-Byrne, 1990). "Decisions about what to teach [women in the prison environment] have been decided largely on the basis of institutional needs as well as notions about what is appropriate work for women" (Moyer, 1984, p. 54).

Conclusion

A wide range of policy recommendations were made by researchers to improve prison-based program quality. It was suggested that educational and vocational programming be complemented with services like career counseling and job placement (Schumacker et al., 1990). Successful vocational programs will provide skills that are in demand for today's job market (Enocksson, 1981; Lawrence et al., 2002) and female facilities should work on providing women with job employment skills that are not for the least paid jobs in the country. Subsequently, discharge planning is an important component for successful post-release outcomes. If the releasee cannot find a job, does not have a place to live, or does not have any community support, the chances of recidivism appear likely with or without previous educational/vocational training.

For female offenders, it would be helpful to complement existing programs with ones that seek to increase levels of self-esteem. Female inmates are plagued by low levels of self-esteem (Pollock-Byrne, 1990) and a sense of powerlessness (Moyer, 1984). Without the self-esteem to generate and uphold smart and confident decisions, most will be unable and ill prepared to make appropriate decisions upon release, particularly when they were powerless to make decisions while incarcerated.

Educational and vocational funding needs to be restored because numerous studies, despite their methodological issues, showed that they are related to successful post-release outcomes. Thus, prison programming has the ability to redirect the life course. Programming is a transition that occurs within the institutional setting and it offers the possibility of altering one's criminal trajectory. The fact that another human being is given skills to help change his/her life is reason enough to keep these programs (Enocksson, 1981). Idleness within the prison system is dangerous and it has the potential of increasing tensions between inmates and staff, and of producing more violence in an already violent atmosphere (Butterfield, 1995).

We are abandoning rehabilitation just as more studies are showing increasing support for the fact that rehabilitation can work (Currie, 1998). In an attempt to save money, congress will be paying for these costs in the long run (Yarbo, 1996). We have the ability to minimize recidivism and in the process reduce incarceration fees, costs to victims, costs to law enforcement, court costs, and reclaim lost income taxes (Harer, 1995). Since education and treatment has never been funded properly, we did not save that much money by eliminating it (Van Voorhis, 1987), but we can save a lot of money by restoring it.

Little research has been conducted on less traditional vocational opportunities behind bars, such as HIV/AIDS peer education programs. Working in an HIV peer education program helps inmates acquire essential employment skills that may lead to an increased adherence to conventionality, subsequently resulting in reduced recidivism and prison disciplinary infractions. With the decrease in traditional programming, less traditional programs take on increased importance, especially in lieu of the programmatic problems in female facilities.

Chapter 5
The Success of HIV Prison-Based Peer Programming

Introduction

The pains of imprisonment for women can be improved by revolutionizing the way we view nontraditional programming in prison. Nontraditional prison-based programming like ACE and CARE provides a multitude of benefits to correctional administrators. Besides the obvious benefit of education, these peer programs allow the women offenders who work for them to obtain marketable job skills, obtain a higher purpose in life, cultivate conventional networks of support, limit the effects of prisonization and maladjustment, and increase levels of institutional success (i.e., decreased disciplinary infractions) and post-release success (i.e., reduced recidivism). ACE and CARE became an inmate's extended family in the prison system. Women adopted a new conventional role while incarcerated and had the system of support necessary to maintain that role when released. ACE/CARE provided these women with genuine friendships that supported their new conventional identities both inside and outside of the prison walls. Within this supportive network, women expressed their emotions in a healthy manner without fear of receiving punishment for emotional outbursts. Older women in the program mentored the younger women, helping them to adjust to their newfound identity, and therefore decreasing the rate of maladjustment. Drawing from social control and life course theories, the evidence cited about the rehabilitative effects of prison programming, and the need for HIV programming in prison, this study showed that peer programs led to successful outcomes for female peers both inside and outside of the penitentiary.

Peer Programming

Peer-based programs provide many advantages to inmates and correctional administration. The benefits of inmate-led peer education are multifaceted: Inmates trust other inmates, speak the same language, have similar backgrounds,

K. Collica, *Female Prisoners, AIDS, and Peer Programs: How Female Offenders Transform Their Lives*, SpringerBriefs in Psychology,
DOI 10.1007/978-1-4614-5110-5_5, © The Author 2013

have complete availability for the population (especially on the weekends when civilian staff is not present), are cognizant of the risky behaviors that occur in prison, and are completely cost effective (Hammett, Harmon, & Maruschak, 1999; US Conference of Mayors AIDS Information Exchange, 1995). Peer participants serve as a liaison between inmates and prison staff, allowing services to be provided more efficaciously (Syed & Blanchette, 2000b). Studies indicate that inmates tend to prefer HIV education conducted by inmate peers (Grinstead, Faigeles, & Zack, 1997).

Peer education in prison reduces initial risky post-release behaviors (i.e., unprotected sexual activity and needle use) (Grinstead, Zack, Faigeles, Grossman, & Blea, 1999). In general, peer education programs prove to be effective in many areas, including, but not limited to, working with those who suffer from mental illness (Barber, 2005). Research generated from Canada highlighted the positive effects of peer-based programming in prison for female offenders. These programs trained female inmates to provide emotional support for one another. Both inmates and prison staff stated that such programs were extremely helpful and beneficial for inmate participants, particularly for the peer themselves (Syed & Blanchette, 2000a, 2000b). Moreover, many peer educators, once released from the prison, were able to obtain paid positions in the field of HIV. "Not only have these programs had a positive impact on those utilizing the service, but the peer educators themselves have gained heightened insight into their lives, empowering them to move beyond their criminal lifestyles" (Devilly, Sorbello, Eccleston, & Ward, 2005). Despite the benefits gained from the implementation of inmate-led peer education, only 13% of state/federal prisons and only 3% of city/county jails (Hammett et al., 1999) used this system. Some staff may feel that peer programs allocate too much power to certain inmates. Peers are often allowed to move throughout the facility to provide educational services and they have movement privileges that other inmates do not have (Clark & Boudin, 1990). There is also the issue of ensuring that peers are adequately trained, supervised, and able to hold confidentiality to the highest of standards, as well as remembering that "peer educators are not substitutes for professionals, but are complimentary" (Devilly et al., p. 237).

Levels of Knowledge

Education is the best preventative tool in the fight against HIV. Few facilities, however, provide all-inclusive programming, such as comprehensive HIV education (CDC, 1996; Hammett et al., 1999) and even fewer ones conduct studies to determine the effectiveness of their programs on inmates (Devilly et al., 2005; Martin, Zimmerman, & Long, 1993). Hammett et al. 1999 defined comprehensive programming to embody "instructor-led education, peer-led programs, pre and posttest counseling and multi-session prevention counseling" (p. 27). Unfortunately, they reported that only 10% of state/federal prisons and only 5% of city/county jail systems offered programs that fit these criteria.

The CDC (1996) cite five cardinal reasons for the implementation of HIV education in prison: (1) There is a high rate of those infected and those at risk for HIV, (2) there are continued risks for transmission during incarceration through both sexual activity and drug activity, (3) these individuals will be released back into the community, (4) there are very high rates of recidivism among this population, and (5) there is the work-ability of providing such programs. It appears that discrepancies between one's level of knowledge about HIV and one's behavior may be attributed to the following factors: (a) the ways in which the education is being presented, (b) the lack of supplementary services (i.e., counseling, testing, etc.), and (c) little or no follow-up services during incarceration and/or once ex-offenders are released back into their community. ACE and CARE are two programs that meet the definition of "comprehensive" or "all-inclusive" programming.

An earlier investigation of ACE was conducted to determine whether subjects experienced increased levels of knowledge as a result of their participation in ACE's HIV curriculum.[1] Women participating in the ACE Program at BHCF were asked to voluntarily participate in a study seeking to understand the effectiveness of prison-based HIV/AIDS programming. This study investigated the levels of knowledge surrounding HIV/AIDS, self-reported precarious behavior leading to an increased risk for HIV infection, and perceptions of future behavior modification based on information/services received from the ACE Program. Pre- and post-test question-naires were utilized as a tool to measure levels of knowledge, risk perceptions, and perceptions of future behavior modification.

Overall, test scores proved to significantly increase from the original pre-test scores ($t = -5.899$, df$= 26$, two-tailed significance $p = 0.000$, 95% *confidence interval*, lower$= -18$ and upper$= -9$) to the post-test scores. The increase in scores showed an association between educational workshops on HIV and an increase in knowledge surrounding HIV directly proceeding the classes (see Fig. 5.1). The most common incorrect answers on both the pre- and post-test were to the follow-ing statements: "It is easier for a woman to infect a man with the AIDS virus than it is for a man to infect a woman," "The AIDS virus is a very easy virus to get," and "It is very likely that a person will get the AIDS virus from a blood transfusion." At the completion of the workshops ($n = 27$), 74% of the women felt that they had learned a great deal of new information. Seventy-seven percent found this informa-tion to be very useful and 75% were glad that they attended these classes. Over half (51%) expressed an interest in receiving more advanced information on HIV/AIDS, 43% desired to attend a support group, and 34% wanted to be an ACE orga-nizational member. Women who knew someone who died as a result of AIDS-related complications and women who reported drug addiction were more likely to

---

[1] This study was conducted by the author in 2002. Data were collected over a 2-month period, covering three sets of HIV workshops. Each group of women received 2 weeks of HIV education. The study yielded a sample size of 35 women for the pre-test and 27 women for the post-test. The questionnaire was a revised version of the National Health Interview Survey AIDS Knowledge and Attitudes Supplement (Kerwin, 1993), which obtains information on general levels of knowledge, transmission behaviors, and common misperceptions in regard to HIV infection.

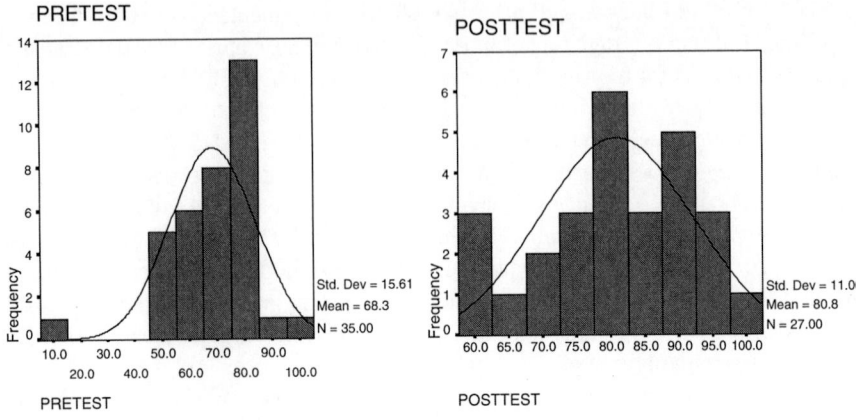

Fig. 5.1 Test Scores—Histogram

score higher on the pre- and post-tests when compared to other subjects. Most women expressed a desire to modify their behaviors based on the information provided to them during the workshop series. It is evident that HIV peer programs are able to provide numerous benefits to prison officials by providing inmates with increased knowledge, accurate risk perceptions, and a cost-effective method of providing educational services.

Methods

Once it was determined that inmate subjects who participated in these programs could increase their knowledge regarding HIV, it was necessary to examine how the programs affected the inmate peers. Therefore, the purpose of the current study was to investigate the benefits for inmates who work in an HIV prison-based peer program, while adding to the criminology literature on female patterns of criminality.[2]

---

[2] See Appendix A for specific hypotheses.

It provided a preliminary understanding of how prison programs affect the processes of criminal desistance and behavioral changes for female inmates. The author hypothesized that women who worked in ACE/CARE obtained stronger social bonds than those female inmates who have not worked for ACE/CARE, subsequently reducing levels of recidivism and institutional disciplinary infractions. Based on social control theory and life course theory, it was hypothesized that women who worked in these programs developed high levels of self-esteem, attachments to conventional others, involvement and commitment to conventional activities, and possessed beliefs in accordance with conventional rules. The strength of these social bonds (an important component of life course theory) determined levels of success both in and out of the correctional facility. The social bonds that developed from working as a peer educator served as a life transition that altered the criminal trajectory. This qualitative study, based on the narratives of 49 female offenders, examined the effects of ACE and CARE, two HIV prison-based peer programs, on inmate peers in NYS.

The sample included (a) women incarcerated in BHCF and TCF who were currently working as peer educators for ACE or CARE, (b) women incarcerated in one of NYS' five female facilities (Albion, Bayview, Beacon, Bedford Hills, or Taconic) who had previously worked as peer educators for ACE/CARE or both programs, and (c) formerly incarcerated women living in the community who, during their incarceration, had worked for ACE, CARE, or both programs. The author collected data from the peers over a 7 month period, from February 2005 to September 2005, yielding a sample of 49 women.[3] Forty-nine percent of the women were formerly incarcerated ($n=24$) and 51% of the women were currently incarcerated ($n=25$). Based upon extensive one-on-one semi-structured interviews with these women, the author utilized a snowball/chain referral sample to obtain additional subjects.[4] Out of 57 women who were identified and located by the author as matching the study's eligibility requirements (i.e., a current/former peer worker for ACE/CARE), seven women declined to participate and one woman, incarcerated at Albion, was unable to be interviewed, yielding a response rate of 86%. Many questions required open-ended responses and yielded in-depth answers that could not easily be reduced to numerical format.[5]

---

[3] The author worked with the women of ACE responsible for implementing the program and Sister Antonia, who was responsible for implementing CARE, to devise a list of all women who worked for both programs. Out of approximately 65 women identified, 49 were interviewed. Women not included were either deported, deceased, or unable to be located. Hence, 75% of all women who worked for both programs participated in this study.

[4] Snowball sampling, though not ideal, was the only way to locate subjects. The DOCCS did not keep records on peer workers.

[5] There are several limitations to the current study. The sample was not a random sample which can pose problems for generalizability. In these types of programs, selection-bias may pose an issue and there was no true control/comparison group. It was not feasible to have another set of women serve as a control in the prison setting. It is difficult to gain approval for prison research. Asking to disturb another group of women was impractical. As a result, the author made in-group comparisons and compared those who worked for ACE/CARE for 1 year/until their release to those who worked for ACE/CARE <1 year. Comparisons were also made between the women responsible for the implementation of the programs and those who began working for the program after their establishment.

The central thesis of social control theory is derived from Travis Hirschi's social bonding/control theory as stated in his book, *Causes of Delinquency* (1969), to measure the strength of bonds between the female peers, the peers and the civilians, and the peers in relation to their overall commitment to the ACE/CARE Program. Many of the questions were modified and are now applicable to prisoners. Questions were borrowed from Sampson and Laub's study (1990) on Life Course Theory, which expanded upon Hirschi's original concept, to measure the strength of job stability, commitment, etc. Others were revised questions from research conducted by Alarid, Burton, and Cullen (2000), Canter (1982), Friedman and Rosenbaum (1988), Lasley (1998), Rankin (1976), Shover, Norland, James, and Thornton (1979), and Rosenbaum (1987). The author devised additional questions to measure social bonding, as well as questions that tapped into specific demographic information and specific information about the women's experiences working in ACE/CARE. On average, interviews took approximately 75 minutes to complete; the shortest interview lasted 35 minutes, while the longest interview lasted 140 minutes. All participation was voluntary (no incentives were allowed) and all interviews were conducted in private. Private rooms were set aside for prison interviews and interviews with formerly incarcerated subjects were conducted in their homes, offices, or another place of their choosing.

The author examined common themes in answers generated by respondents according to the Grounded Theory Approach (Glaser & Strauss, 1967). Responses were recorded in written format by the author (tape recording was prohibited) and transcribed later that day. Categorization of responses and themes continued during transcription. It was believed that the use of both quantitative and qualitative measures would increase the validity of subjects' responses and provide a fuller understanding of the women's experiences.

Demographics of the sample differed slightly from the average NYS prison population. In this sample, whites tended to be overrepresented (33% compared to a 22% rate among the study population), and the age of participants tended to be 4 years older (40 years old compared to an average of 36 years old among the study population) than the average NYS female inmate. Almost all of the women (except for two) had the equivalent to a high school education or higher and 43% of the sample was unemployed prior to their incarceration.

In terms of family status, 59% ($n=29$) had children. The children of these women ranged in age from the youngest being 2 weeks old to the oldest being 39 years old. Out of these 58 children, 36% were 18 years old or younger. Over one-half (61%) of sample participants were unmarried. Many of the subjects (33%) were charged with multiple crimes. In terms of their most serious charge, 49% ($n=24$) were serving time for murder or manslaughter, 31% ($n=15$) were serving time for a drug-related offense, 12% ($n=6$) were serving time for assault, and 2% were serving time for robbery ($n=1$), burglary ($n=1$), kidnapping ($n=1$), or forgery ($n=1$). For subjects who were incarcerated ($n=25$), the average time served at the time of the interview was 11 years 6 months. For subjects who were residing in the community ($n=24$), the average time served in prison was 8 years 8 months.

Findings

Attachment

To measure attachment to ACE/CARE, subjects were asked a series of questions regarding their feelings toward their coworkers, the ACE/CARE civilian staff, and their feelings toward the program in general. Many participants spoke about their ACE/CARE coworkers as being a source of support for them and some referred to their coworkers as "family." In general, the women who worked for ACE/CARE appeared to share a very strong connection with one another and possessed significant attachments. The older members would often act as mentors for the younger members, re-creating a family-like structure. When asked if they felt like working for ACE/CARE was like having an extended family, an overwhelming majority of women (94%) agreed. This feeling of "family" was very important and something that appeared to help them through very difficult periods.

> Many of us are still great friends today. My closest and dearest friends are the women I had worked with in ACE… (Shyone/ACE)[6]

> It was beautiful. We really had a family and some of us were closer than others but we all had each other's back. There was no other place in prison with that type of unity. (Volcano/ACE)

The ACE/CARE civilians were also a part of this "family." They were the few staff members inside of the prison that the women felt that they could trust. These were individuals who would always listen to them and never judge them.

> It was cool, crazy cool. It was just like that. There was never a time that you couldn't talk to them, share with them, or shed a tear with them. I felt that love, which was hard to find in prison. (Blondie/CARE)

The peers experienced a strong relationship with their civilian supervisor. Eighty-nine percent cared a lot about her opinion. Consequently, the women were very aware that their behavior reflected upon the program, their peers, and the civilian staff. Ninety-two percent stated that their supervisor would be upset with them and 69% said their peers would be upset with them if they committed a disciplinary infraction.

> … I respected the people I worked with and some of them were my best friends. I would feel like shit [if I got in trouble]. They placed a lot of trust in me and knew the importance of what I was doing. All of us came from a dysfunctional place and there was an expectation of consistency. If I would have gotten in trouble, it would have stopped the work that I was doing. I needed to keep my shit clean. They respected the work I was doing and they had trust and faith in me that I would excel. (W21/ACE)

Most of the women respected the dedication of the civilian staff and admired their goals, strength, and passion, with 86% maintaining that they served as role models for them.

---

[6] Participants were asked to choose their own code name.

> [I respected them] because of their care and concern about the team and their patience in general. [Supervisor's name] gave hours and hours of herself and didn't even get paid for all of that extra time. (Compassionate/ACE)

> …I looked up to them and I always wanted to be as knowledgeable about HIV and AIDS as they were. (Sky/ACE)

The inclusion of civilian staff was recognized as an integral component of the program. Ninety-four percent of participants stated that the program was better with civilian staff involvement. Most women commented on the fact that civilian staff members were necessary to keep the program "running smoothly." They did not feel that the civilian staff was there to usurp their power within the program. They served as a complement to the inmate staff. Most respondents claimed that the civilian staff were necessary to provide leadership, guidance, support, and provide services that the inmates were unable to provide (i.e., meet with administration, schedule events, make phone calls, etc.).

> [The program] is better because the civilians give some type of structure to the program. Without structure, who will the inmates answer to? Without civilians, we can only do so much. We only have but so much power. We can't answer the phones or make outside contacts. We need civilians. (Enigma/CARE)

Since incarceration can be extremely stressful, particularly for female inmates, who suffer emotionally because of the separation from their family and children, being a part of ACE/CARE assisted in ameliorating these stress inducing factors. Fifty-three percent of the sample stated that the separation from family was the most difficult, particularly being separated from their children and the constant worrying about their well-being. Many of these subjects also had to deal with the loss of a family member while in prison. Other subjects stated that they felt powerless, they hated being locked in, having no freedom and little privacy. Others expressed concern over the inconsistencies in the rules, being dehumanized, having to take orders all of the time, and going in front of the parole board. For the time that the women worked in the program(s), 98% of subjects found support via ACE/CARE and felt that the ACE/CARE peers and civilian staff were very helpful during stressful times in their lives.

The variable of attachment to civilian staff and peers was also measured by asking subjects if they had a lot of respect for the peers and civilians and if they shared their thoughts and feelings with them often. Ninety-two percent stated that they had "a lot" of respect for the civilian staff, only 8% said that had respect for only "some" of the civilian staff. In regard to their coworkers, 65% of respondents stated that they had "a lot" of respect for their peers, while 31% stated they only had respect for "some" of their peers. Most of the women stated that even if they did not like a particular peer, they still possessed the ability to respect her and the work that she was trying to accomplish within the program. ACE/CARE served as a safe emotional outlet for stress. Ninety-four percent shared their feelings with "all" or "some" of the peers and 86% shared "a lot" or "some" of their feelings with the ACE/CARE civilians.

To determine if some peers were more likely than other types of peers to have strong attachments to their coworkers or to the ACE/CARE civilian staff, their answers to questions measuring the variable of attachment were either given a score of one or zero.[7] The highest score a respondent could obtain for both was 14 points, while the lowest score was a zero. In general, levels of attachments were high but comparisons between the groups of women (i.e., those who stayed with the program until their release compared to those who left the program prior to release and those responsible for implementing the program vs. those who started working after the program was established) did not prove to be statistically significant.[8] Overall, the score for attachment to coworkers for both groups was fairly high (mean = 10.6; median = 11; mode = 11). Additionally, the score for attachment to ACE/CARE civilian staff for both groups was very high (mean = 13; median = 13; mode = 14).

Specific questions were asked of participants to measure levels of attachment to the ACE/CARE Program(s). When asked about their job responsibilities within the program, most respondents stated that their main job responsibility was education and counseling (90%). When asked why they decided to work for ACE/CARE, many of the women maintained that they "wanted to help others" (43%), they wanted to educate others and learn more about HIV infection (39%), they had a loved one who had died of AIDS related complications (14%), or they wanted to lessen the stigma associated with being HIV positive (4%).

> I worked for ACE because after I went through the course and I learned that the educator, one of the founders, was HIV positive, I wanted to know more. Once I started, I never left. I have been in the field for 15 years. I went to CARE because this is what I do. It's fulfilling for me. It gives me the chance to be there for somebody else. I can give them a shoulder to cry on. Some people just can't accept their status but I can be there with them to help them cope. (Hopeful/ACE & CARE)

All participants stated that ACE was a positive experience for them (100%), but the reasons they cited varied. Sixty-one percent of the women declared that the most positive aspect of the ACE/CARE program was learning a tremendous amount of information and acquiring skills which they felt would help them to obtain employment upon release, while 28% believed that the work gave their lives meaning because they enjoyed helping others. The rest of the participants believed that the most positive aspect of the program was that it changed the negative views of others (6%), it kept them out of trouble (2%), and they liked working with the other peers (2%).

> It gives your life meaning in here. There are people who live on the outside who have never touched as many lives as we did through ACE. (Purposed/ACE)

Seventy-eight percent of subjects believed their time in prison would have been different if they did not work for ACE/CARE. If they were not involved with ACE/

---

[7] A score of one signified that there was a high to moderate level of attachment, while a score of zero signified that there was a low to no level of attachment. There were 14 questions to measure levels of attachment to coworkers and 14 questions to measure attachment to civilians.

[8] Those who stayed with the program until their release and those responsible for the implementation of the program(s) had slightly higher levels of attachment to their coworkers, the civilians, and the program, than those who did not stay with the program until their release and those who worked for the program after its inception but it was not statistically significant. Specific questions can be located in Appendix B.

CARE, the women believed that their time would have passed more slowly, they would have been in more trouble in the prison setting, they would not have learned cardinal health information, they would have not been able to help others, and they would not have experienced a strong sense of community.

> It gave me a sense of being here, of not just being in prison but building a sense of community. The prison's normative structure is so alienating and ACE allowed us to create great warmth and support, and create a dynamic culture that was not drug oriented or violence oriented, like most prison programs, but caring oriented. It was enormously helpful for me as a long termer to help me build a life here. (Ruby/ACE)

Working for ACE/CARE helped subjects to maintain a positive self-image and provided peers with a higher purpose. It appeared that the perceptions of both inmate population and prison staff had an effect on how the women perceived themselves. These positive perceptions gave the women confidence and made them feel as if they were making a positive difference in the lives of others. Seventy-four percent felt correctional staff perceived them differently than other inmates and 94% felt they were also perceived differently by other inmates. Over one-half of the sample (53%) thought that they were perceived as more dependable, more educated, more respected, or more trustworthy by staff than other inmates. They also felt they were perceived as role models and held to a higher standard than other inmates.

> I was perceived as someone who was serious and doing something meaningful. I was always respected. Except for one officer, I had no problems. I carried myself well and when I entered the units, they knew I was there to do my job. If I said I was going up there to counsel someone, they knew I was up there to counsel and that's it. They knew I wouldn't cause a problem. (Shak/CARE)

Seventy-one percent of subjects believed they were viewed as more knowledgeable, more trustworthy, and more supportive than other inmates. They also felt that they were viewed as role models by other inmates.

> …When they [the inmates] saw me, they would say she works for ACE. She does the workshops. You can talk to her, you can trust her. Many of the women have trust issues but they felt safe talking to us… (Blissful/ACE)

Subjects thought so highly of the program(s) that 90% would recommend ACE/CARE to other inmates interested in working in the field of HIV. The most common reason stated as to why respondents would recommend ACE/CARE to other inmates was due to the tremendous amount of knowledge and marketable job skills that could be gained (55%). All of the women had very high perceptions of how their work was evaluated in ACE/CARE by themselves and by their supervisor.

Different questions were asked of subjects who were incarcerated and subjects who were released to measure levels of attachment to the program once they have/had left prison. Incarcerated respondents strongly desired to maintain some contact with their ACE/CARE coworkers (84%) and the ACE/CARE civilians (96%) upon being released. Ninety-two percent ($n=22$) of releasees kept in contact with their former ACE/CARE peer workers and most (75%) maintained contact with the ACE/CARE civilian staff since their release. For releasees ($n=24$), 88% ($n=21$) worked in an HIV-related position, particularly within the first 6 months of release. At the time of the interview, 75% of releasees were still employed in an HIV-related position. The desire of women to remain in contact with the programs upon release demonstrates strong attachment levels. In order to determine respondents' overall attachment to the program, 13 questions, measuring attachment, were scored accordingly. The highest score one could obtain was 13 points, while the lowest score one could obtain was zero points. Overall, levels of attachment to the program(s) by subjects were fairly high (mean = 11; median = 12; mode = 12).[9]

Commitment

To measure the variable of commitment, participants were asked questions to determine their level of commitment to the ACE/CARE program and their level of commitment to achieving higher educational and vocational aspirations. The first seven questions, which measured commitment to ACE/CARE, were based on a Likert scale, from strongly agree to strongly disagree (see Table 5.1). Respondents were asked to choose the best response to the statement that was being read to them by the author. Based on responses, levels of commitment to ACE/CARE by participants were extremely high.

In addition to personal goals, subjects had goals for the program(s). When asked if there was anything about the program(s) that they would like changed, 63% wanted the programs' existing services expanded, 14% stated they would focus on current staffing issues, and 2% wanted increased funding. Most of the women (90%) believed that working in ACE/CARE helped them or would help them to successfully make the transition from the prison environment to the community. Sixty-three percent of participants stated that the transition was or would be easier because of the knowledge they gained and the skills they acquired. Many believed it would help them or has helped them to obtain employment positions that they would not have otherwise been able to attain. Some stated that the skills they learned and the positive feelings they acquired would be useful in all employment and personal settings.

> … it helped me to put job skills on my resume. I am grateful for the skills I developed, which is what helped me to get a good job. It is always interesting to say that you were part of this program. (Power/ACE & CARE)

> … it would help anyone like myself feel confident about our job marketability. I saw those who left prison with only a high school diploma but because they had their certificate from the CARE office, they were able to get a good job when they went home. CARE also gave us a lot of freedoms and it helped us escape some of the confinement. Unlike the other women,

---

[9] Those who stayed with the program until their release had slightly higher levels of attachment to their coworkers than those who did not stay with the program until their release. These differences proved to be statistically significant (*Mann–Whitney U statistic = 74; Wilcoxon W statistic = 480*). The associated p value of 0.000 was statistically significant at the <0.0005 level. No statistically significant differences existed among those responsible for program implementation. See Appendix B for specific questions.

Table 5.1 Participant commitment to ACE/CARE

Statement	Frequency				Percent				N
	SA	A	D	SD	SA	A	D	SD	
The only reason I worked for ACE/CARE was because I needed a job	0	0	6	43	0	0	12	88	49(100%)
The only reason I worked for ACE/CARE was because I didn't want to work in a low level prison job like a porter	0	0	0	49	0	0	0	100	49(100%)
I feel the skills that I obtained in ACE/CARE have helped/will help me to obtain a good job upon release	32	16	1	0	65	33	2	0	49(100%)
Whatever I did at ACE/CARE, I tried hard	42	7	0	0	86	14	0	0	49(100%)
I really enjoyed the work I was doing in ACE/CARE	44	5	0	0	90	10	0	0	49(100%)
I thought I did really good work in ACE/CARE	39	10	0	0	80	20	0	0	49(100%)
I thought the work I did in ACE/CARE was important	47	2	0	0	96	4	0	0	49(100%)

Percentages may be more or <100% due to rounding

SA strongly agree, A agree, D disagree, SD strongly disagree because we worked for CARE, we were allowed to go on all of the galleries (housing units). Officers would open a room for us during quiet hour to counsel some of the women. We weren't as locked up as the rest of the women. Because of that, we left without feeling so angry and rebellious. The freedom, I believe, helped to alleviate the stress. (Shak/CARE)

All of the women, when asked about their long-term goals, gave very positive responses in terms of educational, professional, and personal aspirations. Goals for this population were strong, thereby augmenting the bond of commitment. Many of the women were determined to complete their college education, others wanted to open their own businesses, own their own homes, or live a peaceful and fulfilling life with their families. In terms of educational aspirations, 31% were in school at the time of the interview. Three were working toward an AA degree, seven toward a BA/BS, two toward a MA, two toward a GED, and one toward a Ph.D. Seventy-one percent were hopeful that they would continue their education in the near future. In terms of ultimate educational goals, 31% wanted a MA/MS/MSW, 20% of the women wanted a BA, 8% wanted CASAC certification, 10% wanted a Ph.D., and 2% wanted certification as a nurse's assistant. In regard to vocational aspirations, 61% stated that they wanted to work in some form of social services. Most of the women chose a position in which they could spend their lives helping disadvantaged populations. To measure their levels of commitment to conventionality, 12 questions asked of participants were scored and compared accordingly.[10] The highest score attainable was 12. The overall score for commitment for all respondents was extremely high (mean = 11; mode = 12; median = 12, with a standard deviation of 0.7922).

Involvement

Participants were asked questions to determine the level of involvement each woman had to conventional activities inside and outside of the penitentiary. In regard to prison life, most of the women had a very high level of involvement in prosocial activities while incarcerated. While employed in ACE/CARE, respondents spent a large quantity of their time with their peer coworkers and the ACE/ CARE civilian staff.

We spent all of our time together when I worked for ACE. We were together a couple of nights a week in IPC. On the weekends we were in the children's center, and many of us also lived together. We could never get away from one another. You have to parole to get away. (Purposed/ACE)

The most common conventional program that respondents were involved with while in prison was school. Eighty-six percent of respondents attended an academic program while incarcerated. Respondents also spent a large quantity of time involved in other types of programming while in prison, such as drug programs, parenting programs, anger management programs, the puppy program, and family violence

---

[10] See Appendix B for scored questions.

programming. While in prison, respondents spent most of their time by themselves (39%), with their friends (33%), or with the ACE/CARE staff (29%).

Releasees were asked questions to measure their level of involvement in the community. Eighty-four percent were employed at the time of the interview. For the three women who were unemployed, one woman stated she was too ill to work, and the other two women had recently moved to another area and were still unable to find employment. Most (18) of the women worked for community-based organizations providing social services, two worked for colleges, and one worked as a waitress. Twenty of the women were happy with their current position and were in their current position for an average of 18 months. Eighteen of the women stated that they liked their current supervisor, 17 of the women planned on staying at their current job for at least one more year, and all employed releasees worked an average of 34 h per week. When asked about their last evaluation, 15 received a favorable evaluation from their supervisor, while 6 women had not worked at their agency long enough to receive a work evaluation. Employed respondents reported that they were late to work or called in sick for work very infrequently.

To measure levels of involvement in conventional activity, hours were computed weekly for how the women spent their time in prison. There are 168 h in a week but inmates are only allowed out of their cells or off of their housing units for approximately 84 h per week, including the time allotted for meals. Respondents were viewed as having a very high level of involvement in conventionality if they spent at least 75% of those hours (63 h) involved in conventional behavior. The hours included in this analysis were hours spent in ACE/CARE, hours spent with ACE/CARE peers outside of work, hours spent in school, additional hours spent on schoolwork, hours spent in other prison programs, and hours spent in religious services. Overall, all respondents spent a very high number of hours per week involved in conventional activities while in prison (mean = 69; median = 67; mode = 86; standard deviation = 28.66). Since a large part of their day was spent involved in conventional programs, most respondents (73%) did not believe that they "had a lot of free time" on their hands while in prison. These women were able to keep extremely busy by being involved in prosocial activity while incarcerated.

For releases, conventional hours included work hours, school hours, additional hours spent on school work, hours devoted to volunteer work, and hours spent with their partner, their children, and their family members. Overall, releasees had a very high number of hours involved in weekly conventional activity (mean = 60; median = 61; mode = 38). The bond of involvement for these women was strong. This finding differs from Hirschi's original study and the subsequent research of other academics who did not find strong evidence to support the bond of involvement in promoting conventional behavior (Agnew, 1985; Burton, 1991; Hirschi, 1969; Torstensson, 1990). With the exception of a few researchers, such as Hindelang (1973), who did find that strong involvement in conventional activities was correlated with reduced rates of delinquency, involvement has typically been the least supported of all the bonds.

Belief

The variable of belief was measured by reading 11 different statements (see Table 5.2). Answers were based on a Likert-scale from strongly agree to strongly disagree. Surprisingly, less than one-half of the women believed that ACE/CARE prevented them from violating prison rules, while others believed they would still obey or still break the same amount of rules no matter where they were working. This finding was very interesting considering most of the women experienced a decrease in prison disciplinary infractions while working in the program(s).

In general, the peers had moderate levels of belief in conventional norms. Most of the women stated that they abided by prison rules and regulations (78%), most agreed that inmates should be held responsible for the crimes they committed (66%) and the prison rules they had broken (76%), most agreed that you should not be dishonest, manipulative, or corrupt in order "to get ahead in life" (64%), and most stated that they had respect for correctional officers (59%) and the police (57%). These percentages, though, were not extraordinarily high. In contrast, most felt that the prison rules that inmates broke during their incarceration were not very serious (67%), and almost one-half (49%) believed that an inmate who left her locker unlocked and was stolen from was just as much to blame as the inmate who stole from her locker (51%). Again, these percentages were not very high. Overall, 11 questions were asked to rate respondents' belief scores; responses were given a score of either one or zero.[11] The highest score one could obtain was 11, while the lowest score was zero. Overall, participants obtained a moderate score on the belief scale (mean=7; median=7; mode=8; standard deviation=2.05). Belief was the least supported of all of the bonds.

Self-esteem

All respondents were asked ten questions to measure levels of self-esteem (see Table 5.3). Questions measuring levels of self-esteem were from the ten-item Guttman self-esteem scale "which has satisfactory reproducibility and scalability (Rosenberg, 1965)," and can predict varying ranges of self-esteem levels (O'Brien, 1985).

To measure levels of self-esteem and make comparisons accordingly, a value was assigned to each of the possible responses.[12] The scale ranged from 0 to 30 points, with 30 points being the highest possible score. Those scoring between 0 and 10 points received a low self-esteem rating, those scoring between 11 and 20 points received a moderate self-esteem rating, and those scoring between 21 and 30 points received a high self-esteem rating. Overall, the study participants had very high levels of self-esteem (mean=26; median=26; mode=28; standard

---

[11] See Appendix B for questions.

[12] See Appendix B for scoring.

Table 5.2 Participants and the bond of "belief"

Statement	Frequency					Percent					
	SA	A	D	SD	DK	SA	A	D	SD	DK	N
I abided by prison rules and regulations	23	15	8	3	0	47	31	16	6	0	49(100%)
I thought it was OK to break prison rules if I could get away with it	8	16	10	15	0	16	33	20	31	0	49(100%)
I couldn't stay out of trouble in prison no matter how hard I tried	3	1	13	32	0	6	2	27	65	0	49(100%)
Most inmates should not be blamed for the crimes they committed	4	8	18	14	5	8	16	37	29	10	49(100%)
Most crimes really do not hurt anyone	1	5	14	28	1	2	10	29	57	2	49(100%)
Most inmates should not be blamed for the prison rules they have broken	0	9	24	13	3	0	18	49	27	6	49(100%)
Most of the rules that inmates break while in prison are not that serious	8	25	11	2	3	16	51	22	4	6	49(100%)
An inmate who leaves her locker unlocked and is stolen from is just as much to blame as the inmate who steals from her locker	6	19	12	12	0	12	39	25	25	0	49(100%)
I have a lot of respect for correction officers	5	25	12	4	3	10	51	25	8	6	49(100%)
I have a lot of respect for the police	5	23	12	5	4	10	47	25	10	8	49(100%)
To get ahead you have to do some things which are not right	1	14	17	14	3	2	29	35	29	6	49(100%)
I would have violated more prison rules if I didn't work for ACE/CARE	8	14	18	9	0	16	29	37	18	0	49(100) %

Percentages may be more or <100% due to rounding

SA strongly agree, A agree, D disagree, SD strongly disagree, DK donot know

Table 5.3 Participants and Rosenberg's self-esteem scale

Statement	Frequency				Percent				N
	SA	A	D	SD	SA	A	D	SD	
On the whole, I am satisfied with my life	18	23	6	2	37	47	12	4	49(100%)
At times I think I am no good at all	2	8	9	30	4	16	18	61	49(100%)
I feel I have a number of good qualities	45	4	0	0	92	8	0	0	49(100%)
I am able to do things as well as most other people	38	9	1	1	78	18	2	2	49(100%)
I feel I do not have much to be proud of	1	2	7	39	2	4	14	80	49(100%)
I certainly feel useless at times	1	10	15	23	2	20	31	47	49(100%)
I feel that I am a person of worth, at least on an equal plane with others	43	6	0	0	88	12	0	0	49(100%)
I wish I could have more respect for myself	1	5	15	28	2	10	31	57	49(100%)
All in all I am inclined to feel that I am a failure	0	3	10	36	0	6	20	74	49(100%)
I take a positive attitude toward myself	37	11	0	1	76	22	0	2	49(100%)

Note. Percentages may be more or <100% due to rounding
SA strongly agree, *A* agree, *D* disagree, *SD* strongly disagree

deviation = 4.01). In terms of their self-esteem rating, 94% received a rating of "high" self-esteem, 6% received a rating of "moderate" self esteem, and 0% received a rating of "low" self-esteem.

Institutional Success

Institutional success was measured in terms of disciplinary infractions and the number of tickets an inmate received during the course of her incarceration. To determine if working in ACE/CARE had an effect on the rate of tickets incurred, respondents were asked to report on the total number of tickets they received prior to and during the time they were employed with ACE/CARE. Inmates were asked how they would describe their own disciplinary history, if they perceived themselves as a disciplinary problem and if they felt that others perceived them as a disciplinary problem. Eighty-five percent of participants rated their disciplinary history as good or excellent and 92% did not perceive themselves as a disciplinary problem. Eighty-six percent did not believe others saw them as a disciplinary problem. When asked if they received any tickets during the course of their incarceration, 80% of the women said they received one or more tickets, while only 20% stated they never received any tickets. In NYS, tickets are based on a tier system, with tier ones being the least serious infractions and tier threes being the most serious infractions. Most of the tickets received were for minor infractions.

> I had four tickets, two tier ones and two tier twos. One tier one was before ACE for having a teddy bear and one tier two, which was during ACE, was for altering my skirt. After ACE, I had two tier twos for refusing a pat frisk by a male officer. (Jada/ACE). I received one ticket. I disobeyed a direct order but it was a long time ago. The officer wrote me up for talking to somebody behind the grill (the gate). I didn't know that the grill was the gate. The only grill I know is for hamburgers and hotdogs. I was new and didn't know. This was in 84 when I first got there. So because I didn't understand him, I didn't move, and he wrote me the ticket. He should have said gate." (Air/ACE)

In looking at the effect that ACE/CARE had on rates of disciplinary infractions among participants, more than one-half of participants (51%) had a decrease in the number of tickets they received after joining ACE/CARE. Forty-seven percent did not experience any changes, as the rate of infractions among this group was low before working for ACE/CARE, and only one woman, who was a severe disciplinary problem and fired from her position, experienced an increase in tickets incurred. On average, the women had received 5.17 tickets prior to working for ACE/CARE (0.59 tier ones, 4.10 tier twos, 0.52 tier three) and they only received, on average, 1 ticket (0.95) during the time they worked for ACE/CARE (0.19 tier ones, 0.70 tier twos, 0.10 tier threes). This shows a substantial decrease in the rate of infractions after joining the ACE/CARE staff. Overall, when utilizing a paired samples t test, the decrease in the rate of disciplinary infractions proved to be statistically significant ($t = 2.918$, $df = 46$, two-tailed significance $p = 0.005$, 95% confidence interval = 1.30–7.11), illustrating a correlation between working for an HIV prison-based peer education program and better institutional conduct.

For those women who received tickets (80% of the sample), most of the infractions (53%) were for minor rule violating behaviors, such as smoking, illegal exchange (i.e., giving something or receiving something from another inmate), contraband (i.e., mostly hygiene items or food items that they were not allowed to have), disobeying a direct order or being out of place. Twenty-four percent were for assault and/or fighting or a "DG" (i.e., degenerative act, meaning having physical contact with another inmate), and one woman, who had the highest rate of disciplinary infractions, received most of her tickets for dirty urines.

In comparison to national rates of disciplinary infractions among all inmates, the rate of infractions among ACE/CARE inmates (1 per year) was lower than the national average (1.5 per year) (Stephan, 1989). In comparison to all female offenders, the rate of infractions among ACE/CARE peers (1 per year) was one-half of the national average for female inmates (2 per year) (Stephan, 1989).

For many tier two and tier three infractions, inmates can be punished by being "keep locked." When an inmate is on keep-lock status, they are locked in their cell for 23 out of 24 h per day. Forty-seven percent of the sample population reported being on keep-lock status; however, most were locked prior to working for ACE/CARE. The rate of keep lock decreased substantially after an inmate began working for ACE/CARE and these results proved to be statistically significant ($t=2.289$, $df=19$, two-tailed significance $p=0.034$, 95% confidence interval 0.1627–3.6373).

Twenty-two percent ($n=11$) of the women reported serving SHU (Special Housing Unit) time during their incarceration. SHU, which is strict solitary confinement, is located in a separate part of the facility at BHCF, and inmates are locked in a cell for 23 out of 24 h a day and receive minimal to no privileges. Eight of these women served their SHU sentence(s) prior to working for ACE/CARE, one served a SHU sentence during the time she worked for ACE for having a fight with another inmate, and one inmate served a SHU sentence both before and during the time she was employed with ACE, which was also for fighting. Two women reported being placed in administrative segregation, but this was after they had left the ACE Program.

Post-release Success

All 25 releasees experienced high rates of success. Almost all of the releasees ($n=21$) were employed full-time at the time of their interview. Only three of the releasees were not working. One woman was not working due to illness and the other two women recently moved. They were both employed full-time prior to moving. Eighteen of the women worked for community-based organizations providing social services such as HIV related services, mental health services, and substance abuse services, two worked for colleges, and one worked as a waitress. Twenty of the women were happy with their current position and had been in their current position for an average of 18 months. Moreover, six of the women were employed in supervisory positions (i.e., program coordinators, program managers, and program directors).

On average, releasees were living in the community for 5 years (median=4 years; mode=10 years) since their release from prison, ranging from the shortest time out of prison at 1 year and the longest time out of prison at 15 years. Only one of the releasees was arrested since leaving prison. Nonetheless, her transgression was quite minor and she was not violated by her parole officer. *Tyler* (ACE) explained what happened:

> I was arrested over Christmas time on a trespassing charge. The whole thing was ridiculous. I went to the projects to see my friend but she wasn't there. As I was leaving, the police stopped me and said that because my friend wasn't there, no one could verify that I was actually visiting her, so they arrested me on a trespassing charge.[13] I couldn't fucking believe it. They just wanted the overtime and they didn't want to be out patrolling the projects in the snow. I had a shitty public defender so I pled guilty to a misdemeanor and received three days community service.

The women were also asked to report any law violating or parole violating behavior that escaped the attention of the authorities or their parole officer. Nine of the women reported committing parole violations and/or engaging in illegal behaviors. Two of the women admitted to drinking alcohol occasionally, two admitted to drinking alcohol occasionally in addition to missing curfew, two admitted to having smoked marijuana on one or two occasions, one admitted to missing her curfew, one admitted to leaving the jurisdiction, and one admitted to stealing when she was first released. None of the releasees, however, were ever sent back to prison for a new arrest.

Two of the incarcerated participants, who had worked for CARE and were released, had returned to prison on a technical violation. Both women were violated for leaving the jurisdiction. *Pandora* was violated for absconding from her work release program. She stated that she had become involved in a very unhealthy relationship with a man whom she later married. She believed that this failed relationship contributed to her leaving her program. The second woman, *Determined*, was violated by her parole officer when she went to Pennsylvania to visit her ill father. Technically, nine releasees could have been violated, even though their violating behavior, for the most part, was minor in nature. In most cases, the majority of the women in the sample population managed to maintain a law-abiding lifestyle and achieved a high level of post-release success.

In general, out of the 26 women who were released from prison after working for ACE/CARE, two returned to prison for a technical violation and were awaiting release at the time of the interview ("Determined" is now home) and one was rearrested for trespassing but was not sent back to prison. Therefore, the official recidivism rate for this population is at 12% ($n=3$) (see Fig. 5.2). To lend further credibility to these results, the author conducted a follow-up interview with releasees 1 year later and none of the releasees had returned to prison. In addition, three of the incarcerated subjects were released in the past year. Since release, they have not committed any technical or legal violations and all three gained purposeful

---

[13] It is illegal to be on public housing grounds if you do not live in the building or if you are not visiting someone who lives in the building. If you are visiting and no one is home to verify your visit, you can be arrested for trespassing.

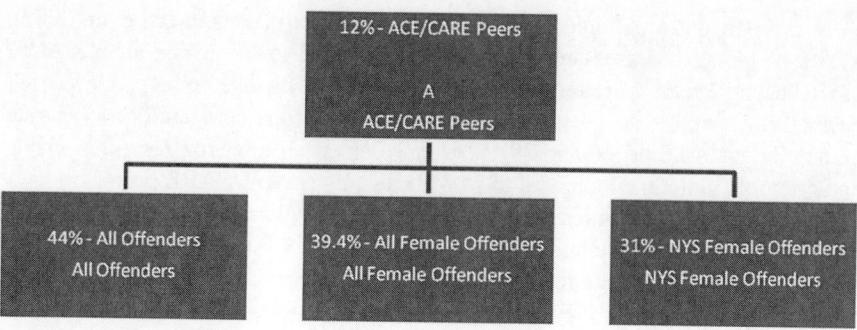

Fig. 5.2 Recidivism rates

employment. On average, the ACE/CARE releasees were living in the community for 5 years. The unofficial recidivism rate for this population, including the nine women who admitted to committing violations but were not caught for their behavior, is at 46%.

When compared to official rates of recidivism nationally (Langan & Levin, 2002), ACE/CARE peers had a much lower rate of recidivism when compared to all offenders released from American prison facilities (12% vs. 44%). They were also less likely than other American female inmates to face additional prison time after release for either committing a new crime or for committing a parole violation (12% compared to 39.4%, respectively) (Langan & Levin).

ACE/CARE peers seemed to have lower rates of recidivism than other female releasees in NYS. In 2002, 31% of women in NYS were returned to prison for parole violations (Staley, 2003), while only 8% of ACE/CARE peers were returned. The same rates were also found in 1999 after a 3-year follow-up study of NYS inmates. Female releasees returned to prison at a rate of 30% (Kellam, 1999), compared to an 8% rate among ACE/CARE peers. There are no national statistics or state statistics on unofficial rates of recidivism; hence, a comparable analysis could not be conducted.

When rates of recidivism are further divided between rearrest rates and reimprisonment rates due to parole violations or the commission of new crimes, the disparities in the numbers are even more impressive. In a report compiled by the Bureau of Justice Statistics (Langan & Levin, 2002), national rates of recidivism for all offenders were operationalized through four different means: rearrested for a new criminal offense, reconvicted for a new criminal offense, resentenced to prison for a new criminal offense, and reimprisoned for a new criminal offense and/or parole violation. Within 3 years of release, 67.5% of releasees were rearrested compared to a 4% rate among ACE/CARE peers; 46.9% were reconvicted compared to a 4% rate among ACE/CARE peers; 25.4% were resentenced to prison for a new offense compared to a 0% rate among ACE/CARE peers; and 51.8% were resentenced to prison for a new crime and/or parole violation compared to an 8% rate among ACE/CARE peers.

In comparison to national female rates of recidivism (Langan & Levin, 2002), 57.6% of female releasees were rearrested compared to a 4% rate among ACE/CARE peers; 39.9% were reconvicted compared to a 4% rate among ACE/CARE peers; 17.3% were resentenced to prison for a new crime compared to a 0% rate among ACE/CARE peers; and 39.4% were resentenced to prison for a new crime and/or parole violation compared to an 8% rate among ACE/CARE peers.

In comparison to figures compared by the New York State Department of Correctional Services (Kellam, 1999), within 3 years, 7% of female releasees and 13% of male releasees were resentenced to prison for the commission of a new crime compared to a 0% rate among ACE/CARE peers, and 23% of female releasees and 28% of male releasees were returned to prison for a parole violation compared to a rate of 8% among ACE/CARE peers. Although the ACE/CARE release sample is quite small, it is evident that these peers have a substantially lower rate of recidivism than all other offenders, irrespective of the way in which recidivism is measured.

Civilians

The author interviewed three former ACE/CARE civilian supervisors to obtain a different perspective about HIV prison-based peer programs. The civilians stated that ACE and CARE are important programs, not only because of the education it provides but also because of the humanity it provides in an inhumane environment. When asked about the difficulties in managing such programs, the civilians cited problems working effectively within the rules and regulations of the prison system. It was difficult to provide innovative programming in a place where security issues take priority over treatment. The civilians stated that their best experience in these programs was working with the peer educators. It brought them a tremendous amount of joy to watch the women transform their lives and to see the women excel at something that they loved doing. For many of the women, it was the first time they had ever had a job and it was something that brought them an incredible amount of self-respect and recognition. In regard to the most challenging part of maintaining a peer education program, the civilians stated that finding responsible women to work as peers was difficult, in addition to trying to provide comprehensive services in a highly regimented environment.

National Survey

Although peer programs are successful, most facilities are not utilizing them for educational or rehabilitative purposes. The author conducted a national survey, which was mailed to all 50 states' Department of Correctional Services main administrative headquarters and the Federal Bureau of Prisons. This enabled the author to obtain information on the extent of such programs in the USA (see Table 5.4). All 50 states and the federal government responded to the survey, yielding a response rate of 100%.

Table 5.4 The National Survey on HIV Prison-Based Peer Programs

Department	No. of prisons	No. of inmates	No. of female inmates	Rate of HIV infection	Mandatory testing	HIV peer program
Alabama	32	27,487	1,857	1%	Yes	Yes
Alaska	13	3,299	330	1%	No	No
Arizona	10	32,570	2,786	0.5%	No	No
Arkansas	18	12,547	758	1%	Yes	Yes
California	89	163,939	11,476	Unknown	No	No
Colorado	23	20,144	1,915	1%	Yes	No
Connecticut	18	17,933	1,312	Unknown	No	No
Delaware	10	6,787	514	2%	No	Yes
Florida	59	81,975	5,299	4%	Yes	Yes
Georgia	42	49,551	3,196	2%	Yes	No
Hawaii	8	3,918	528	0.4%	No	No
Idaho	15	6,284	696	0.4%	Yes	No
Illinois	27	43,012	1,439	1%	No	Yes
Indiana	34	22,544	1,977	0.5%	Yes	No
Iowa	9	8,580	767	0.4%	No	Yes
Kansas	8	8,966	646	0.4%	No	Yes
Kentucky	13	12,285	730	Unknown	No	No
Louisiana	11	19,400	900	Unknown	No	Yes
Maine	6	2,004	117	0.5%	No	Yes
Maryland	26	24,000	900	4%	No	No
Massachusetts	18	9,749	760	3%	No	Yes
Michigan	42	50,123	2,165	1%	Yes	Yes
Minnesota	8	8,333	490	0.6%	No	No
Mississippi	35	19,266	1,646	1%	Yes	No
Missouri	21	30,768	2,516	1%	Yes	No
Montana	3	3,599	419	0.2%	No	No
New Hampshire	4	2,500	150	0.5%	Yes	No
Nebraska	11	4,075	367	0.4%	Yes	No
Nevada	9	11,372	878	1%	Yes	No
New Jersey	14	25,499	1,397	5%	No	Yes
New Mexico	5	6,172	572	0.5%	No	No
New York	70	66,000	3,000	5%	No	Yes
North Carolina	76	35,756	2,466	2%	No	No
North Dakota	4	1,200	Under private contract	0.3%	Yes	No
Ohio	33	44,040	2,948	1%	Yes	No
Oklahoma	17	23,670	2,422	0.5%	Yes	Yes
Oregon	12	12,780	948	0.4%	No	No
Pennsylvania	27	40,185	1,805	2%	No	Yes
Rhode Island	8	3,243	263	3%	Yes	No
South Carolina	29	22,807	1,555	2%	Yes	No
South Dakota	7	3,075	290	1%	No	No
Tennessee	12	19,394	1,157	1%	Yes	No
Texas	96	15,077	12,022	2%	Yes	Yes

(continued)

Table 5.4 (continued)

Department	No. of prisons	No. of inmates	No. of female inmates	Rate of HIV infection	Mandatory testing	HIV peer program
Utah	2	6,004	515	0.6%	No	No
Vermont	9	1,544	144	Unknown	No	Yes
Virginia	52	31,983	1,983	1%	No	No
Washington	16	17,000	1,000	1%	No	No
West Virginia	11	3,838	320	0.3%	No	No
Wisconsin	40	21,825	1,329	1%	No	No
Wyoming	4	1,222	133	0.5%	Yes	No
Feder BOP	114	182,255	12,358	1%	Yes	No

[a]*Note.* Rate of infection percentages rounded to the nearest hundredth
[b]Numbers for private facilities were not reported

In total, the results of the national survey included 1,280 facilities and 1,427,279 inmates, of which 1,331,118 were male inmates, and 96,161 were female inmates. When asked how education was provided to their inmate population, most stated that the medical staff provided such services (75%; $n = 24$), followed by civilian staff (16%; $n = 5$), the Department of Health (6%; $n = 2$), and one state (3%; $n = 1$) distributed literature on HIV for inmates to read. For those states that provided HIV prison-based peer programming, 6 states had between 1 and 5 programs, 6 states had between 6 and 11 programs, 1 state had between 11 and 15 programs, 1 state had between 16 and 20 programs, 2 states had between 26 and 30 programs, and 2 states had over 30 programs. Texas had the most programs, with 43 HIV peer programs for their inmates. With regard to peer programs, 83% provided discharge planning services, 78% provided confidential HIV testing, 22% provided anonymous testing, 44% provided professional trainings, 72% provided educational workshops, 33% provided resource/health fairs, 28% provided other special events and 83% provided HIV counseling. Not all of the facilities within the same state provided the same services (see Table 5.5).

In 1999, Hammett et al. found that only 10% of state/federal prisons offered what they termed "comprehensive programming," which was defined as "instructor-led education, peer-led programs, pre and posttest counseling and multi-session prevention counseling (p. 27)," and only 3% of state/federal prison systems offered inmate-led peer education. In the current national survey, 18% of state/federal prisons claimed to have an HIV peer education program, a slight increase from the 1999 study, but these numbers are still incredibly small and such programs are not represented in most of our American facilities. Even for those states that had HIV peer education programs, these programs were not available in all of their facilities. Since private prisons were not included in the survey, it is unknown how inmates contracted to privately managed facilities are receiving HIV education.

States that did not have HIV peer programs appeared apprehensive about placing inmates in such a high status position and they were afraid that inmates would break confidentiality. Other facilities stated they did not have the money to fund such programs, they did not have an HIV peer education program because their rates of HIV infection were extremely low, or they had implemented alternative ways of educating their inmates.

Table 5.5 HIV peer programs and their services

State	No. of peer programs (No. of prisons)	Discharge planning (No. of prisons)	Confidential testing (No. of prisons)	Anonymous testing (No. of prisons)	Professional trainings (No. of prisons)	Educational workshops (No. of prisons)	Health or resource fair (No. of prisons)	Annual events (No. of prisons)	HIV counseling (No. of prisons)	Other (No. of prisons)
Alabama	19	X(19)			X(19)				X(19)	
Arkansas	6	X(1)	X(6)			X(4)		X(6)	X(6)	
California	28	X(28)	X(28)						X(28)	
Delaware	10	X(10)	X(10)			X(10)			X(10)	
Florida	6	X(6)	X(6)			X(6)			X(6)	
Illinois	26	X(26)	X(26)			X(26)	X(26)	X(26)		
Iowa	5	X(5)	X(5)			X(5)			X(5)	
Kansas	8	X(8)	X(8)	X(8)	X(8)	X(8)	X(8)	X(8)	X(8)	
Louisiana	11	X(11)	X(11)		X(11)	X(11)	X(11)		X(11)	
Maine	1	X(1)	X(1)	X(1)	X(1)	X(1)	X(1)		X(1)	
Massachusetts	7	X(7)	X(7)						X(7)	
Michigan	2	X(2)	X(2)						X(2)	
New Jersey	4	X(4)				X(4)			X(4)	
New York	45	X(45)	X(45)	X(45)	X(45)	X(45)	X(2)	X(2)	X(45)	Support groups; HIV Hotline
Oklahoma	3									
Pennsylvania	10					X(10)		X(10)		
Texas	57	X(57)	X(57)	X(57)	X(57)	X(57)	X(57)		X(57)	
Vermont	3	X(3)	X(3)	X(3)					X(3)	

For those states that did have HIV peer programming, none of the programs, except for ACE/CARE in NYS, had outside civilian staff members based in the facility on a full-time basis. This may be why ACE/CARE has enjoyed so much success over the last 21 years. It is much easier for staff to gain the trust of the inmates when they are in the facility all of the time. It also has the added benefit of civilians becoming more familiar with the prison administration. This will prove to be especially beneficial when HIV programs propose new program initiatives If civilian staff are deemed trustworthy by prison administration, and trust only comes with time, they might be given more lead way in terms of managing the program. Staff members who are "in and out" of the facility are less likely to be trusted by both inmates and prison officials and they are less likely to gain a complete understanding of the prison environment, the inmates that they are working with, and the prison administrators that they are technically working for. Having a program office and a full-time program staff offers the program a greater degree of stability.

Implications

The implications of this research are considerable. This research provided evidence that HIV prison-based peer programming had numerous beneficial effects. First, in terms of its impact on theory and the criminological literature, the author studied a particular aspect of corrections that has yet to be examined. Previous research showed that HIV prison-based peer programs provide increased levels of knowledge surrounding HIV and helped to create accurate risk perceptions among participants (see Collica, 2002; 2006), but researchers have ignored the unintended benefits of these programs, which are the benefits derived for the peers themselves (Collica, 2010). A few researchers have pointed to the beneficial effects of peer programs on the peers themselves, but the evidence was anecdotal at best (Collica, 2010). Neglecting this important area led to a gap in the knowledge-base surrounding peer education programs in prison. This study helped to bridge the gap between prior research and anecdotal evidence by shedding light on a neglected issue.

Second, this study adds to our understanding of social control theory and life course theory, and its impact in explaining paths of desistance for the female offender. Most of the literature focusing on recidivism has focused on male offenders (Harm & Phillips, 2001), and the desistance process for female offenders still remains a mystery (Katz, 2000). It is evident from this study that HIV prison-based peer programs is one way to provide female peers with strong social bonds, even while incarcerated. The quality and strength of the bonds that developed from working for ACE/CARE helped to redirect the female criminal's pathway, aided in altering her criminal trajectory, and assisted in the process of criminal desistance.

Third, this research complements penology literature which has focused on the beneficial effects of educational and vocational programs as tools in the rehabilitative process for criminal offenders. Traditional prison programming, which is academically or vocationally based, has been found to assist in the reintegrative process

(Correctional Educational Bulletin, 2002) by reducing recidivism (Canestrini, 1993; Clark, 1991; Gerber & Fritsch, 1995; Harer, 1995; MacDonald, 1995; Taylor, 1992), by increasing levels of self-esteem (Roundtree, Edwards, & Dawson, 1982; Tewksbury & Vito, 1994), and by promoting communication with positive civilian staff members who will help to reinforce law-abiding norms and values (Gaes, Flanagan, Motiuk, & Stewart, 1999; Harer, 1995; Taylor, 1993). Little research has been conducted on less traditional vocational programs like ACE/CARE and the research that was previously conducted did not focus on the benefits achieved by the peers who worked for such programs. This research shows that inmates who worked in an HIV prison-based peer program can achieve the same effects derived from traditional prison programs. ACE/CARE helped to develop essential employment skills, increased levels of self-esteem, opened up lines of communication with positive civilian staff members, and aided in the reintegrative process. All of these factors subsequently reduced disciplinary infractions by promoting prosocial behavior in prison and by allowing the peers to obtain meaningful and purposeful employment upon release. It also led to reduced rates of recidivism.

In lieu of the harsh restrictions placed upon felons in our country (i.e., disenfranchisement, limitations on access to employment opportunities, public housing, public assistance, or federal/state aid for college programming, termination of parental rights, etc.) (see Travis, 2002), ACE/CARE provides a way for female offenders to be successful after release (Collica, 2006; 2010). One of the fields that appear to be wide open to ex-offenders is the field of HIV/AIDS. Many community-based organizations that provide HIV-related services, particularly in the New York City area, have hired ex-offenders to provide outreach, case management, and educational and supportive services to their clients, most of whom are also recently released from prison or jail. ACE/CARE provided the women with a great opportunity to acquire the skills they needed in prison to attain entry-level positions upon release in the field of public health. For many of the releasees, this was the beginning of a successful career or at least an initial way for them to support themselves financially when they first returned home.

ACE/CARE provided these women with a higher purpose in life and it enabled them to adopt the role of the "wounded healer" or "professional ex" (Maruna, 2001), which helped them in maintaining a conventional lifestyle. They were able to use their work in ACE/CARE to bring together their two identities; the old criminal identity and the new law-abiding identity (Lofland, 1969; Nouwen, 1972). These women did not have to be ashamed of their past because they were able to utilize it as a tool to help others. This new way of looking at themselves provided new insight into their past and allowed them to turn something 'bad' into something "good," thereby aiding the process of criminal desistance.

Fourth, this research adds to the literature on prisonization and rates of maladjustment among female inmates. The way inmates adapt to the prison environment and the role they adopt while incarcerated to ameliorate the pains of imprisonment (Heffernan, 1972; Schrag, 1944; Sykes & Messinger, 1960) can have a direct effect on rates of disciplinary infractions and recidivism. As a survival mechanism, female inmates have been known to re-create family inside of the prison (Giallombardo,

1966), but recent evidence shows that the nature of the play family is evolving and has decreased in recent years (Genders & Player, 1990; Propper, 1982). If the way that females tend to adapt to the prison environment is under transformation, then this may change rates of maladjustment inside of the prison environment. ACE/CARE has been shown to provide the peers with new roles. ACE/CARE is not only their family, it enables them to cultivate strong conventional relationships while in prison. ACE/CARE is a new prison subculture, albeit, a positive one and one that encourages conventional change. Considering that ACE/CARE became an inmate's extended family while in the prison system, the women were able to adopt new conventional roles while incarcerated and have the system of support necessary to maintain those roles when released. This network of support protects them from adhering to many of the norms inherent in the inmate subculture, it decreases the chances of prisonization, and it prevents maladjustment, which can effect prison infractions and rates of recidivism. These women are viewed as role models and their new identities are supported and encouraged by their coworkers and the ACE/CARE civilian staff. These women were very cognizant of the effect that their behavior would have the overall success of the program, and for the most part, they were not willing to engage in behavior that could result in prison disciplinary action; most were unwilling to jeopardize their position or jeopardize the overall success of the program.

Fifth, in regard to research methodology, this study has implications for conducting research with female offenders. The author found the use of open ended questions particularly helpful in eliciting in-depth and detailed responses from the female participants. Since many questions on the interview schedule were open-ended, it encouraged the women to answer in their own words. The author was surprised to see that this "openness" set the tone for the entire interview and had a bearing on the closed-ended responses as well. The women became comfortable talking to the researcher and even when a participant was asked to choose a specific response to a closed-ended question or statement, they almost always provided additional information. This was very helpful upon analysis when attempting to gain a fuller understand of these women, their experiences, and their feelings.

Sixth, the use of snowball sampling as a data collection method worked very well with this population. Since inmates often have a distrust of staff, this enabled the author to speak to women who normally would not have spoken to her. The women were happy to refer the author to other peers and many releasees spent considerable time making phone calls and sending e-mails to these other peers on the author's behalf. Several of the women stated that they would not have spoken to the author if they were not referred by one of their peers. Another factor, which appeared to help in the interviewing process, was that many of the peers were familiar with the author and the work she has performed in the prisons. This certainly lent credibility to her study and increased the bond of trust between researcher and interviewee. It is also believed that gender played a significant role in the interviewing process. The women would probably not have been as open with a male researcher. The author received several responses from the respondents prefaced with things like, "you're a woman, you know" or "As a woman I am sure you can understand".

Seventh, in regard to policy implications, the success of such programs should prove that there is not only a need to maintain funding for existing programs but also a need to expand funding to implement and enhance HIV prison programs in all facilities, particularly for female inmates (Collica, 2007). Female facilities suffer from a paucity of prison programming, and since their needs tend to be more diverse and more substantial than the needs of their male counterparts, increasing and expanding such programming are essential. If female inmates continue to be trained in pink-collar employment, they will be unable to support themselves or their children upon release. Female inmates trained in HIV peer education can and will be able to obtain substantial employment opportunities in major metropolitan cities upon release.

These benefits not only affect inmates but also the prison administration, the Division of Parole, the community, and various CBOs. Correction officials have an incentive to implement or maintain current peer education programs since inmates can obtain higher success levels while in prison by having reduced rates of disciplinary infractions. Given that the programs are subsidized by CBOs, they are completely cost effective for correctional departments and they provide invaluable services. Until a cure is found, HIV continues to be a chronic illness plaguing inmates in our correctional institutions. If education can serve as a means for prevention, our prisons will undoubtedly save tremendous costs in medical care and related services. Moreover, for those individuals who contract a multidrug resistant strain of HIV, the costs of treating subsequent opportunistic infections will be substantial. Inmates engage in risky behaviors behind bars, and without adequate knowledge about safer sex and drug using practices, they could become infected with HIV or Hepatitis, and for those who are already HIV infected, they could be exposed to other drug resistant strains of the virus. Prisons have the opportunity to prevent further transmission of the virus and the opportunity is found within the services of peer education programs.

The community and the Division of parole will benefit from such programs because when inmate peers transition from prison to the community, there will be a lower rate of recidivism. This has a positive impact on parole supervision and community safety, and if we can prevent women from returning to prison, we stand to save a tremendous amount of money on recommitment fees. Women, who leave prison and are educated about HIV transmission, may be less likely to place themselves or others at risk for infection, and they may be more likely to spread this information to friends and family, reinforcing the message of HIV prevention in the community.

Last, CBOs that support such programs will have initial empirical data that prison-based peer programs are correlated with degrees of success, which may enable them to attain or sustain funding from state, local, and federal funding sources. Many states are facing a budget crisis, and in lieu of the current recession, we can only expect further cutbacks, particularly in regard to correctional programming and AIDS-related services. Many CBOs in the NYC area have already lost contractual AIDS funding, including WPA that lost some of its funding from the AIDS Institute for ACE and CARE. Without adequate funding, services will dwindle and everyone will inevitably pay the costs.

Conclusion

This study, based on quantitative and qualitative analyses, was able to show that working in an HIV prison-based peer program was correlated with high rates of institutional and post-release success. Peers received reduced rates of prison disciplinary infractions while working for ACE/CARE, and releasees, who previously worked for ACE/CARE, maintained a low rate of recidivism. In total, the ACE/CARE female peers had high levels of attachment to conventionality, high levels of commitment to conventionality, high levels of involvement in conventionality, moderate levels of belief in conventionality, and high levels of self-esteem. The peers learned marketable job skills. Their work in ACE/CARE provided the peers with a higher purpose; all the women believed that they were making a difference in the lives of others. However, upon conducting group comparisons (i.e., those peers who stayed with ACE/CARE until they were released vs. those peers who left that program prior to release, and those peers responsible for the creation of ACE/CARE vs. those peers who were not responsible for the creation of ACE/CARE), minimal differences were found between the groups, showing that one's status or one's time within such programs does not have an appreciable effect on benefits derived; these programs can prove to be successful for all peers. Moreover, for most peers, ACE/CARE was utilized as a transitional factor which enabled them to modify their criminal trajectory.

Appendix A

Hypotheses One, Two, Three, and Four

1. Inmates working in a peer education program, particularly those women who worked in ACE/CARE for over a period of one or until they were released will
   (a) Have stronger attachments inside and outside of the prison system to individuals also engaging in conventional activities.
   (b) Have a deeper commitment to conventional activities.
   (c) Have acquired a deeper involvement in conventional activities.
   (d) Hold more conventional beliefs.
   (e) Have higher levels of self-esteem.
   (f) Be more successful both in and out of prison

than those who left the program prior to one year or prior to their release.[1]

2. Those women who were instrumental in the creation and implementation of the ACE/CARE Programs will
   (a) Have stronger attachments inside and outside of the prison system to individuals also engaging in conventional activities.
   (b) Have a deeper commitment to conventional activities.
   (c) Have acquired a deeper involvement in conventional activities.
   (d) Hold more conventional beliefs.
   (e) Have higher levels of self-esteem.
   (f) Be more successful both in and out of prison

than those women who were not initially responsible for the creation of the program.

3. Those inmates employed in ACE/CARE will have a lower recidivism rate than most female inmates in the USA in general, and in New York State in particular.
4. Although peer programs are successful, most facilities are not utilizing them for educational or rehabilitative purposes.

---

[1] No one left the program before 1 year.

K. Collica, *Female Prisoners, AIDS, and Peer Programs: How Female Offenders Transform Their Lives*, SpringerBriefs in Psychology, DOI 10.1007/978-1-4614-5110-5, © The Author 2013

Appendix B

Questions below provided data for the quantitative analysis. Additional questions were asked for the qualitative analysis. The full interview schedule can be located in the following work: *From Incarceration to Rehabilitation: Transitions that Transcend the Criminal Trajectory* (2006). Unpublished Doctoral Dissertation, City University of New York, NY by the author.

Attachment to Coworkers

The first question, "How would you describe your relationship with your peer workers," was an open-ended question. Answers were given a score of one if they were positive in tone. Answers such as "great," "good," and "we were like family, would be considered positive responses, while negative responses were given a score of zero. The next two questions, "How many of your coworkers seemed to care about how successful you were while in prison" and "How many of your coworkers seemed to care about how successful you would be after being released from prison," were recorded on a Likert-type scale from "all" to "none." Answers such as "all," "almost all," and "many" would generate a score of one, while answers such as "few" and "none" would generate a score of zero. The fourth question asked, "What kind of work did your coworkers expect from you." Answers such as "excellent," and "good" received a score of one, while answers such as "fair," "poor," and "no one cared" received a score of zero. The fifth through seventh questions, "Did you care about what your coworkers thought of you," "Would you say that you had a lot of respect for your coworkers," and "Did you share your thoughts and feelings with your ACE/CARE coworkers," included answers of "a lot" and "some" which scored a rating of one, while answers like "not much" and "not at all" received a rating of zero. The eighth to the eleventh questions were measured on a Likert scale from "a lot" to "not at all." These questions included, "Did you find your coworkers to be helpful to you during stressful times," "Were your coworkers some of your best friends," "Would your coworkers have stuck by you if you got into trouble," and "Do you respect your

K. Collica, *Female Prisoners, AIDS, and Peer Programs: How Female Offenders Transform Their Lives*, SpringerBriefs in Psychology, DOI 10.1007/978-1-4614-5110-5, © The Author 2012

coworkers' opinions about the important things in life." Respondents who answered "all" or "most" received a rating of one, while those who answered "some" or "none" received a rating of zero. The last three questions included only two answers. If respondents answered "yes" they received a score of one, if they answered "no" they received a score of zero. These questions included, "Did you feel that working for ACE/CARE was like having an extended family," "Would your coworkers in ACE/CARE be upset with you if you committed a disciplinary infraction," and "Would it bother you if your coworkers were upset with you." The highest score a respondent could obtain was 14 points, while the lowest score was a zero.

Attachment to ACE/CARE Civilian Staff

There were 14 questions to measure levels of attachment to the ACE/CARE civilian staff. The first question asked, "How would you describe your relationship with the civilian ACE/CARE staff." Positive responses were given a score of one, while negative responses were given a score of zero. All participants, except for two, responded positively providing answers such as "wonderful," "caring," "they were like family," and "great." The next two questions asked, "How many of the ACE/CARE civilians seemed to care about how successful you were while in prison" and "How many of the ACE/CARE civilians seemed to care about how successful you would be after you were released from prison." Answers such as "all," "almost all," and "many," were given a score of one, while answers like "few" or "none" were given a score of zero. The fourth question asked, "What kind of work did the ACE/CARE civilians expect from you." Answers such as "excellent" and "good" received a rating of one, while answers such as "fair," "poor," and "no one cared" received a rating of zero. The next three questions asked, "Did you care about what your ACE/CARE supervisor thought of you," "Would you say that you had a lot of respect for the ACE/CARE civilian staff," and "Do/did you share your thoughts and feelings with the ACE/CARE civilian staff." Those who answered "a lot" or "some" received one point; those who answered "not much" or "not at all" received zero points. The eighth and ninth questions gave respondents one point for answers like "all" and "most," while zero points were given for answers like "some" and "none". These two questions included, "Did you find the ACE/CARE civilian workers to be helpful to you during stressful times" and "Do you respect the ACE/CARE civilians' opinions about the important things in life." The next four questions that measured attachment to civilian staff were based on "yes" or "no" responses, where a response of "yes" received a rating of one point and a response of "no" received a rating of zero points. Questions included, "Would your ACE/CARE supervisor have stuck by you if you got into trouble," "Would your ACE/CARE supervisor be upset with you if you committed a disciplinary infraction," "Would it bother you if your supervisor was upset with you," and "Do you feel that the ACE/CARE civilian staff were able to serve as role models for you." The last question asked if the peers felt the program was better or worse with civilian staff involvement. Those who stated "better" received one point for their answer, while those who answered "worse," "don't know," or "depends," received zero points for their answer. The highest score a respondent could obtain was 14 points, while the lowest score was a zero.

Attachment to ACE/CARE

To determine respondents' overall attachment to the program, 13 questions, measuring attachment, were scored accordingly. The highest score one could obtain was 13 points, while the lowest score one could obtain was zero points. The first question, "Why did you decide to work for ACE/CARE," was an open-ended question and coded for content. Those who replied with positive answers, such as they wanted to help others, they wanted to make a difference, and they wanted to gain more knowledge, were given a score of one, while those with negative responses were given a score of zero. The next eight questions, "Do you feel that working for ACE/CARE has been a positive experience for you," "Do you think your time in prison would have been different if you had not worked for ACE/CARE," "While working in these programs, do you feel that you were perceived differently than other inmates by prison staff," "While working in these programs, do you feel that you were perceived differently by your peers than other inmates," "Would you recommend ACE/CARE to other inmates interested in working in the field of HIV," "Did you/Do you plan to work for ACE/CARE until your release," "Do you plan on working within the field of HIV upon your release/Since your release have you worked in any positions in the field of HIV," and "Do you feel you can contact the ACE/CARE civilian staff for support upon release/on the outside," were based on "yes" or "no" answers. Respondents were given one point for "yes" answers and zero points for "no" answers. Questions ten and eleven asked, "How would you evaluate your work within the ACE/CARE program" and "How did your supervisor evaluate your work within the ACE/CARE program." Subjects were given a rating of one point for answers such as "excellent" and "good, while those who answered "fair" or "poor" were given zero points. The last two questions measuring attachment to the program asked, "Do you plan on keeping in contact with your ACE/CARE coworkers/Do you keep in contact with any of your former ACE/CARE coworkers" and ""Do you plan on keeping in contact with any of the ACE/CARE civilian staff/Do you keep in contact with any of the former ACE/CARE civilians." Respondents were given one point for answering "all," "most," and "some," and zero points for answering "none."

Commitment

The first seven questions were based on a Likert scale from strongly agree to strongly disagree and included statements such as, "The only reason I worked for ACE/CARE was because I needed a job," "The only reason I worked for ACE/CARE was because I didn't want to work in a low low-level prison job like a porter," "I feel the skills I obtained in ACE/CARE have helped/will help me obtain a good job upon release", "Whatever I did at ACE/CARE, I tried hard," "I really enjoyed the work I was doing in ACE/CARE," "I thought I did really good work in ACE/CARE," and "I thought the work I did in ACE/CARE was important". For the first two statements, respondents were given a score of one point if they answered "strongly disagree" or "disagree," but were given zero points if they answered "strongly agree", "agree," or "don't know." For the last five statements, respondents were given a score of one point, if they answered "strongly agree," or "agree," and zero points for answers like "don't know," "disagree" and "strongly disagree."

Respondents were also asked, "How much schooling do you eventually hope to obtain," "What type of career do you aspire to eventually have," "What are your long-term goals," and "Who, if anyone, serves as a role model to you and why." Respondents were given one point if they stated that they had educational/vocational aspirations, if they established long-term goals for themselves, and if they had someone who served as a role model for them. Respondents who stated they did not plan to go back to school, did not plan to go back to work, or did not have any planned goals received a score of zero. Lastly, if respondents answered "yes" to the following question, "Do you feel that working in ACE/CARE has helped you/or will help you successfully transition from prison to the community," they received one point; if they answered "no," they receive zero points.

Involvement

Hours were computed for time spent involved in conventional activity (i.e., programs, work, family, etc.) while in prison and upon release.

Belief

Questions asked included: "I thought it was OK to break prison rules if I could get away with it," "I couldn't stay out of trouble in prison no matter how hard I tried," "Most inmates should not be blamed for the crimes they committed," "Most crimes really do not hurt anyone," "Most inmates should not be blamed for the prison rules they have broken," "Most of the rules that inmates break while in prison are not that serious," "An inmate who leaves her locker unlocked and is stolen from is just as much to blame as the inmate who steals from her locker," and "To get ahead you have to do some things which are not right." If the participant strongly agreed or agreed they received a score of one. If they strongly disagreed, disagreed, or they stated that they did not know, they received a score of zero. Concomitantly, if they strongly agreed or agreed with the following statements: I abided by prison rules and regulations," "I have a lot of respect for correctional officers," and "I have a lot of respect for the Police," they received a score of one. If they strongly disagreed, disagreed, or stated that they did not know, they received a score of zero.

Self-esteem

To measure levels of self-esteem and make comparisons accordingly, a value was assigned to each of the possible responses. The author assigned three points to each favorable item the subject strongly agreed with, two points to each favorable item the subject agreed with, one point for each favorable item the subject disagreed with, and zero points for each favorable item the subject strongly disagreed with. These items included the following: "On the whole, I am satisfied with my life," "I feel I have a number of good qualities," "I am able to do things as well as most other people," "I feel that I am a person of worth, at least on an equal plane with others," and "I take a positive attitude toward myself." Accordingly, the author also assigned three points to each unfavorable item that the respondent strongly disagreed with, two points to each unfavorable item that the subject disagreed with, one point to each unfavorable item that the subject agreed with, and zero points for each unfavorable item that the respondent strongly agreed with. These items included: "At times I think I am no good at all," "I feel I do not have much to be proud of," "I certainly feel useless at times," "I wish I could have more respect for myself," and "All in all I am inclined to feel that I am a failure." Thirty was the highest possible score.

References

ACE (AIDS Counseling and Education Program). (1998). *Breaking the walls of silence: AIDS and women in a New York State maxium-security prison*. Woodstock and New York: Overlook Press.

Act Up/NY. (1990). *Women, AIDS and activism*. Cambridge, MA: South End Press.

Agnew, R. (1985). Social control theory and delinquency: A longitudinal test. *Criminology, 23*(1), 47–61.

AIDS.gov. (2012). *US statistics*. Retrieved from http://www.aids.gov/hiv-aids-basics/hiv-aids-101/overview/statistics/

Akers, R. (1997). *Criminological theories: Introduction and evaluation* (2nd ed.). Los Angeles: Roxbury Publishing Company.

Alarid, L., Burton, V., & Cullen, F. (2000). Gender and crime among felony offenders: Assessing the generality of social control and differential association theories. *Journal of Research in Crime and Delinquency, 37*(2), 171–199.

Andrews, D., & Kiessling, J. (1980). Program structure and effective correctional practices: A summary of the CaVIC research. In R. Ross & P. Gendreau (Eds.), *Effective correctional treatment*. Toronto: Butterworths.

Applegate, B., Cullen, F., & Fisher, B. (1997). Public support for correctional treatment: The continuing appeal of the rehabilitative ideal. *The Prison Journal, 77*(3), 237–258.

Atchley, R., & McCabe, P. (1968). Socialization in correctional communities: A replication. *American Sociological Review, 33*(1), 774–785.

Audeh, T. (1995, June). For New York inmates, class of '95 is last to get tuition. *New York Times,* A14.

Austin, R. (1978). Race, father-absence, and female delinquency. *Criminology, 15*(4), 487–504.

Barber, C. (2005, April 26). A healing journey, from Harvard to the homeless shelters. *New York Times,* p. F.6.

Beckett, K. (1997). *Making crime pay: Law and order in contemporary American politics*. New York, NY: Oxford University Press.

Bell, R., Conard, E., & Suppa, R. (1984). The findings and recommendations of the national study on learning deficiencies in adult inmates. *Journal of Correctional Education, 35*(4), 129–136.

Benson, M. (2002). *Crime and the life course: An introduction*. Los Angeles: Roxbury Publishing Company.

BJS. (2012). *Recidivism*. Retrieved from http://bjs.ojp.usdoj.gov/index.cfm?ty=tp&tid=17.

Block, C., Blokland, A., & Nieuwbeerta, P. (2007). *Life-span offending trajectory of women, ages 12 to 72*. Paper presented at the American Society of Criminology Conference Annual Meeting, pp. 1–21.

Bonta, J., Pang, B., & Wallace-Capretta, S. (1995). Predictors of recidivism among incarcerated female offenders. *The Prison Journal, 75*(3), 277–294.

K. Collica, *Female Prisoners, AIDS, and Peer Programs: How Female Offenders Transform Their Lives*, SpringerBriefs in Psychology, DOI 10.1007/978-1-4614-5110-5, © The Author 2013

Bowker, L. (1981). Gender differences in prisoner subcultures. In L. Bowker (Ed.), *Women and crime in America* (pp. 409–419). New York, NY: Macmillan Publishing Co., Inc.

Brandon, A. (1998). *Perceptions of the vocational educational program in the NYS DOCS 1998.* Albany, NY: New York State Department of Correctional Services.

Brinkley-Rubenstein, L., & Cornett, M. (2010). *Is mandatory HIV testing in prisons a violation of prisoners' rights?: An examination of the existing prison testing policies.* Vanderbilt Law School Health Law Society/Vanderbilt Center for Health Policy: The Health Law and Public Policy Forum.

Brown, M., & Bloom, B. (2009). Reentry and renegotiating motherhood: Maternal identity and success on parole. *Crime and Delinquency, 55*, 313–336.

Brown, B., & Spevacek, J. (1971). Disciplinary offenses and offenders at two differing correctional institutions. *Corrective Psychiatry and Journal of Social Therapy, 17*(4), 48–56.

Burton, V. (1991). *Explaining adult criminality: Testing Strain, differential association, and control theories.* Unpublished dissertation, University of Cincinnati

Burton, V., Cullen, F., Evans, T., Alarid, L., & Dunaway, R. (1998). Gender, self-control, and crime. *Journal of Research in Crime and Delinquency, 35*(2), 123–147.

Butterfield, F. (1995, July 16). Idle hands within the devil's own playground. *New York Times*, 3 sec 4.

Canestrini, K. (1993). *Follow-up study of industrial training program participants 1993.* Albany, NY: New York State Department of Correctional Services.

Canter, R. (1982). Family correlates of male and female delinquency. *Criminology, 20*(2), 149–167.

Cao, L., Zhao, J., & Van Dine, S. (1997). Prison disciplinary tickets: A test of the deprivation and importation models. *Journal of Criminal Justice, 25*(2), 103–113.

Casey-Acevedo, K. (2001). The effect of time on the disciplinary adjustment of women in prison. *International Journal of Offender Therapy and Comparative Criminology, 45*(4), 489–497.

Casey-Acevedo, K., & Bakken, T. (2003). Women adjusting to prison: Disciplinary behavior and the characteristics of adjustment. *Journal of Health and Social Policy, 17*(4), 37–60.

Caspi, A., & Bem, D. (1990). Personality continuity and change across the life course. In L. Pervin (Ed.), *Handbook of personality* (pp. 549–575). New York, NY: Guilford Press.

Caspi, A., Elder, G., & Herbener, E. (1990). Childhood personality and the prediction of life course patterns. *In Straight and Devious Pathways from Childhood to Adulthood.* (ed. Robins, L., & Rutter, M.). New York:Cambridge University Press, 13–35.

CDC. (1996). HIV/AIDS education and prevention programs for adults in prisons and jails and juveniles in confinement facilities – United States, 1994. *JAMA, 275*(17), 306–1307.

CDC (1999). Women and AIDS statistics. *World* (102), 1. http://www.ncbi.nlm.nih.gov/pubmed/11366916.

CDC (2001). HIV and AIDS – United States, 1981–2000. *MMWR Weekly, 50* (4) [Online]. Available from http://www.cdc.gov/mmwr/preview/mmwrhtml/mm5021a2.htm.

Chesney-Lind, M. (1986). Women and crime: The female offender. *Signs, 12*(1), 79–96.

Chesney-Lind, M. (1989). Girls' crime and woman's place: Toward a feminist model of female delinquency. *Crime and Delinquency, 35*(1), 5–29.

Chesney-Lind, M. (1991). Patriarchy, prisons, and jails: A critical look at trends in women's incarceration. *The Prison Journal, 71*(1), 51–67.

Chesney-Lind, M., & Rodriguez, N. (1983). Women under lock and key: A view from the inside. *The Prison Journal, 62*(2) 47–64.

Clark, D. (1991). *Analysis of return rates of the inmate college program participants.* Albany, NY: New York State Department of Correctional Services.

Clark, J., & Boudin, K. (1990). Struggles for Justice Community of women organize themselves to cope with the AIDS crisis: A case study from Bedford Hills Correctional Facility. *Social Justice, 17*(2), 90–109.

Clemmer, D. (1940). *The prison community.* New York, NY: Holt, Rinehart & Winston.

Collica, K. (2002). Levels of knowledge and risk perceptions about HIV/AIDS among female inmates in New York State: Can prison-based HIV programs set the stage for behavior change? *The Prison Journal, 82*, 101–124.

Collica, K. (2006). *From incarceration to rehabilitation: Transitions that transcend the criminal trajectory.* Unpublished doctoral dissertation, City University of New York, NY

Collica, K. (2007). The prevalence of HIV peer programming in American prisons. *Journal of Correctional Health Care, 13*(4), 278–288.

Collica, K. (2010). Surviving Incarceration: Two prison-based peer programs build communities of support for female offenders. *Deviant Behavior, 31*(4), 314–347.

Conly, C. (1998). *The Women's Prison Association: Supporting women offenders and their families.* Washington, D.C.: National Institute of Justice. Retrieved from: https://www.ncjrs.gov/txtfiles/172858.txt.

Correctional Educational Bulletin. (2001). Correctional Education Association releases more results from recidivism study. *Correctional Educational Bulletin, 4*(11), 1–3.

Correctional Educational Bulletin. (2002). National study reaffirms education reduces inmate recidivism. *Correctional Educational Bulletin, 5*(6), 1–2.

Cotten-Oldenburg, N., Jordan, B., Martin, S., & Kupper, L. (1999). Women inmates' risky sex and drug behaviors: Are they related? *The Journal of Drug and Alcohol Abuse, 25*(1), 129–149.

Covington, J. (1985). Gender differences in criminality among heroin users. *Journal of Research in Crime and Delinquency, 22*(4), 329–353.

Cranford, S., & Williams, R. (1998, December). Critical issues in managing female offenders. *Corrections Today, 60*(7), 130–134.

Cullen, F., & Gendreau, P. (1989). The effectiveness of correctional rehabilitation: Reconsidering the 'nothing works' debate. In L. Goodstein & D. Mackenzie (Eds.), *The American prison: Issues in research and policy* (pp. 23–44). New York, NY: Plenum.

Currie, E. (1998). *Crime and punishment in America.* New York, NY: An Owl Book Henry Holt and Company.

Daly, K. (1995). Looking back, looking forward: The promise of feminist transformation. In B. R. Price & N. J. Sokoloff (Eds.), *The criminal justice system and women* (2nd ed., pp. 443–457). New York, NY: McGraw-Hill, Inc.

DeBell, J. (2001). The female offender: Different…not difficult. *Corrections Today, 63*(1), 56–61.

Des Jarlais, D., & Friedman, S. (1988). The psychology of preventing AIDS among intravenous drug users. *American Psychologist, 43*(11), 865–870.

Devilly, G., Sorbello, L., Eccleston, L., & Ward, T. (2005). Prison-based peer-education schemes. *Aggression and Violent Behavior, 10*, 219–240.

Dobash, R., Dobash, R. E., & Gutteridge, S. (1986). *The imprisonment of women.* New York, NY: Basil Blackwell.

Dolan, K., Lowe, D., & Shearer, J. (2004). Evaluation of the condom distribution program in South Wales Prisons, Australia. *The Journal of Law, Medicine and Ethics, 32*(1), 124–128.

Eaton, M. (1993). *Women after prison.* Philadelphia, PA: Open University Press.

Edwards, D. (2010, May 20). Segregating HIV positive inmates is medically unjustified and hinders rehabilitation. *Huff Post.* Retrieved from http://www.huffingtonpost.com/sexual-justice/segregating-hiv-positive_b_580860.html.

Elder, G. (1985). Perspectives on the life course. In G. Elder (Ed.), *Life course dynamics* (pp. 23–49). Ithaca, NY: Cornell University Press.

Elder, G. (1986). Military times and turning points in men's lives. *Developmental Psychology, 22*(2), 233–245.

Elder, G. (2000). The life course. *In Encyclopedia of Sociology, Volume 3.* (ed. Borgatta, E., & Montgomery, R.). New York: Macmillian Reference, 1614–1622.

Enocksson, K. (1981). Correctional Programs: A review of the value of education and training in penal institutions. *Journal of Offender Counseling, Services and Rehabilitation, 5*(1), 5–18.

Farabee, D. (2002). Reexamining Martinson's critique: A cautionary note for evaluators. *Crime and Delinquency, 48*(1), 189–192.

Farrington, D., Loeber, R., & Van Kammen, W. (1990). Long-term criminal outcomes of hyperactivity – impulsivity – attention deficit disorder and conduct problems in childhood. In L. Robins

& M. Rutter (Eds.), *Straight and devious pathways from childhood to adulthood* (pp. 62–81). New York, NY: Cambridge University Press.

Farrington, D., & West, D. (1995). Effects of marriage, separation, and children on offending by adult males. In: Z. Blau (Series Ed.) & J. Hagan (Vol. Ed.), *Current perspectives on aging and the life cycle.* (Vol. 4, pp. 249–281). New York, NY: Jai Dress Inc.

Feinman, C. (1983). An historical overview of the treatment of incarcerated women: Myths and realities of rehabilitation. *The Prison Journal, 62*(2), 12–26.

Flanagan, T. (1983). Correlates of institutional misconduct among state prisoners. *Criminology, 21*(1), 29–39.

Flanagan, T. (1980). Time served and institutional misconduct: Patterns of involvement in disciplinary infractions among long-term and short-term inmates. *Journal of Criminal Justice, 8*(5), 357–367.

Fox, J. (1984). Women's prison policy, prisoner activism, and the impact of the contemporary feminist movement: A case study. *The Prison Journal, 64*(2), 15–36.

Friedman, J., & Rosenbaum, D. (1988). Social control theory: The salience of components by age, gender, and type of crime. *Journal of Quantitative Criminology, 4*(4), 363–381.

Gaes, G., Flanagan, T., Motiuk, L., & Stewart, L. (1999). Adult correction treatment. In M. Tonry & J. Petersilis (Eds.), *Prisons.* Chicago: University of Chicago Press.

Genders, E., & Player, E. (1990). Women lifers: Assessing the experience. *The Prison Journal, 70*(1), 46–57.

Gerber, J., & Fritsch, E. (1995). Adult academic and vocational correctional education Programs: A review of recent research. *Journal of Offender Rehabilitation, 22*(1/2), 119–142.

Giallombardo, R. (1966). *Society of women: A study of a woman's prison.* New York, NY: John Wiley & Sons, Inc.

Gibbens, T. (1984). Borstal Boys after 25 years. *British Journal of Criminology, 24*(1), 49–62.

Glaser, B. G., & Strauss, A. L. (1967). *The discovery of grounded theory: Strategies for qualitative research.* Chicago: Aldine Publishing.

Gondles, J. (1998). Addressing the needs of female offenders. *Corrections Today, 60*(7), 6.

Goodstein, L., & Wright, K. (1989). Inmate adjustment to prison. In L. Goodstein & D. Mackenzie (Eds.), *The American prison: Issues in research and policy* (pp. 229–251). New York, NY: Plenum.

Goord (Commissioner), G. S. (2001). Goord responds to Amnesty report. *DOCS Today, 10*(5), 4.

Graham, J., & Bowling, B. (1995). *Young people and crime* (Vol. 145). London: Home Office

Greenfeld, L. A., & Snell, T. L. (2000). *Women offenders.* Bureau of justice statistics special report. Washington, DC: BJS. Retrieved from http://bjs.ojp.usdoj.gov/content/pub/pdf/wo.pdf.

Greer, K. (2000). The changing nature of interpersonal relationships in a women's prison. *The Prison Journal, 80*(4), 442–468.

Griffin, M. M., Ryan, J. G., Briscoe, V. S., & Shadle, K. M. (1996). Effects of incarceration on HIV infected individuals. *Journal of the National Medical Association, 88*(10), 639–644.

Grinstead, O., Faigeles, B., & Zack, B. (1997). The effectiveness of peer HIV education for male inmates entering state prison. *Journal of Health Education, 28*(6), 31–37.

Grinstead, O., Zack, B., Faigeles, B., Grossman, N., & Blea, L. (1999). Reducing postrelease HIV risk among male prison inmates: A peer led intervention. *Criminal Justice and Behavior, 26*(4), 453–465.

Hagan, J., Simpson, J., & Gillis, A. (1979). The sexual stratification of social control: A gender-based perspective on crime and delinquency. *British Journal Of Sociology, 30,*(1), 25–38

Hammett, T., Harmon, P., & Maruschak (1999). *1996–1997 update: HIV/AIDS, STDs, and TB in correctional facilities.* Washington, DC: National Institute of Justice

Harer, M. (1995). *Prison education program participation: A test of the normalization hypothesis.* Washington, DC: Federal Bureau of Prisons Office of Research and Evaluation.

Harlow, C. (2003). *Education and correctional populations.* Bureau of justice statistics special report. Washington, DC: US Department of Justice

Harm, N., & Phillips, S. (2001). You can't go home again: Women and criminal recidivism. *Journal of Offender rehabilitation, 32*(3), 3–21.

Harrison, L., Butzin, C., Inciardi, J., & Martin, S. (1998). Integrating HIV – Prevention strategies in a therapeutic community work-release program for criminal offenders. *The Prison Journal, 78*(3), 232–243.

Heffernan, E. (1972). *Making it in prison: The square, the cool, and the life.* New York, NY: Wiley-Interscience.

Henrichson, C., & Delaney, R. (2012). *The price of prisons. What incarceration costs taxpayers. Center on sentencing and corrections.* New York, NY: Vera Institute of Justice.

Hewitt, J., Poole, E., & Regoli, R. (1984). Self-reported and observed rule breaking in prison: A look at disciplinary response. *Justice Quarterly, 1*(3), 437–447.

Hindelang, M. (1973). Causes of delinquency: A partial replication and extension. *Social Problems, 20*, 471–487.

Hirschi, T. (1969). *Causes of delinquency.* Berkley: University of California Press.

Holmberg, S. (1996). The estimated prevalence and incidence of HIV in 96 large US metropolitan areas. *American Journal of Public Health, 86*(5), 642–654.

Human Rights Watch. (2004). *No second chance: People with criminal records denied access to public housing.* New York: Human Rights Watch.Retrieved from: http://www.hrw.org/sites/default/files/reports/usa1104.pdf.

Humphrey, E. (1987). *Review of the literature on female security issues.* State of New York Department of Correctional Services Office of Classification and Movement and Division of Program Planning Research and Evaluation

Hunsinger, I. (1997). Austin MacCormic and the education of adult prisoners: Still relevant today. *Journal of Correctional Education, 48*(4), 160–165.

Irwin, J., & Cressey, D. (1962). Thieves, convicts, and the inmate culture. *Social Problems, 10*(2), 142–155.

JAMA HIV/AIDS Information Center (1999). *HIV infection and AIDS.* Available from http://www.ama-assn.org/special/hiv/support/infect.htm

Jensen, G. (1977). Age and rule-breaking in prison: A test of sociocultural interpretations. *Criminology, 14*(4), 555–566.

Jensen, G., & Eve, R. (1976). Sex differences in delinquency. *Criminology, 13*(4), 427–448.

Jensen, G., & Jones, D. (1976). Perspectives on inmate culture: A study of women in prison. *Social Forces, 54*(3), 590–603.

Johnson, R. (1979). *Juvenile delinquency and its origins.* Cambridge: Cambridge University Press.

Jones, R. (1993). Coping with separation: Adaptive responses of women prisoners. *Women and Criminal Justice, 5*(1), 71–97.

Katz, R. (2000). Explaining girls' and women's crime and desistance in the context of their victimization experiences. *Annual Review of Sociology, 6*(6), 633–660.

Kellam, L. (1999). *1999 releases: Three year post release follow-up.* Albany, NY: New York State Department of Correctional Services.

Kerwin, J. (1993). *Questionnaire design research laboratory: Cognitive testing of the 1993 NHIS AIDS knowledge and attitudes supplement* (Working Paper Series No. 4). US Department of Health and Human Services.

Kessler, R., & McLeod, J. (1984). Sex differences in vulnerability to undesirable life events. *American Sociological Review, 49*(5), 620–631.

Klein, D. (1973). The etiology of female crime: A review of the literature. In B. R. Price & N. J. Sokoloff (Eds.), *The criminal justice system and women (1995)* (2nd ed., pp. 3–30). New York, NY: McGraw-Hill Inc. (pp. 30–53).

Knepper, P. (1990). Selective participation, effectiveness, and prison college programs. *Journal of Offender Counseling, Services and Rehabilitation, 14*(2), 109–135.

Koons, B., Burrow, J., Morash, M., & Bynum, T. (1997). Expert and offender perceptions of program elements linked to successful outcomes for incarcerated women. *Crime and Delinquency, 43*(4), 512–532.

Koski, D. (1998). Vocational education in prison: Lack of consensus leading to inconsistent results. *Journal of Offender Rehabilitation, 27*(3/4), 151–164.

Kruttschnitt, C., & Krmpotich, S. (1990). Aggressive behavior among female inmates: An exploration study. *Justice Quarterly, 7*(2), 371–389.

LaGrange, R., & White, H. (1985). Age differences in delinquency: A test of theory. *Criminology, 23*(1), 19–45.

Lahm, K. (2000). Equal or equitable: An exploration of educational and vocational program availability for male. *Federal Probation, 64*(2).

Lance-McCullough, M., Tesoriero, J., Sorin, M., & Stern, A. (1994). HIV infection among New York State female inmates: Preliminary results of a voluntary counseling and testing program. *The Prison Journal, 73*(2), 198–219.

Langan, P., & Levin, D. (2002). *Recidivism of prisoners released in 1994*. Bureau of justice statistics special report. Washington, DC: US Department of Justice.

Lanier, M., & Paoline, E. (2005). Expressed needs and behavioral risk factors of HIV-positive inmates. *International journal of Offender Therapy and Comparative Criminology, 49(5)*, 561–573.

Larson, J., & Nelson, J. (1984). Women, friendship, and adaptation to prison. *Journal of Criminal Justice, 12*(6), 601–615.

Lasley, J. (1998). Toward a control theory of white-collar offending. *Journal of Quantitative Criminology, 4*(4), 347–362.

Laub, J., Nagin, D., & Sampson, R. (1998). Trajectories of change in criminal offending: Good marriages and the desistance process. *American Sociological Review, 63*, 225–238.

Laub, J., & Sampson, R. (1993). Turning points in the life course: Why change matters to the study of crime. *Criminology, 31*(3), 301–325.

Lawrence, S., Meors, D., Dubin, G., & Travis, J. (2002). *The practice and promise of prison programming*. Washington, DC: Urban Institute Justice Policy Center.

Leger, R. (1987). Lesbianism among women prisoners: Participants and nonparticipants. *Criminal Justice and Behavior, 14*(4), 448–467.

Lewis, A. (1994, September 16). Crime and politics. *The New York Times*, A31

Lillis, J. (1994). Prison education programs reduced. *Corrections Compendium, XIX*(3), 1–4.

Linden, R., & Perry, L. (1982). The effectiveness of prison education programs. *Journal of Offender Counseling, Services and Rehabilitation, 6*(4), 43–57.

Lindquist, C. (1980). Prison discipline and the female offender. *Journal of Offender Counseling, Services, and Rehabilitation, 4*(4), 305–318.

Linton, J. (1998) Inmate education makes sense. *Corrections Today, 60* (3).

Lipton, D., Martinson, R., & Wilks, J. (1975). *The effectiveness of correctional treatment: A survey of treatment evaluation studies*. New York, NY: Praeger.

Long, G., Sultan, F., Kiefer, S., & Schrum, D. (1984). The psychological profile of the female first offender and the recidivist: A comparison. *Journal of Offender Counseling, Services, and Rehabilitation, 9* (1/2), 119–123.

Lofland, J. (1969). *Deviance and identity*. New Jersey, NJ: Prentice Hall.

Lord, E. (1995). A prison superintendent's perspective on women in prison. *The Prison Journal, 75*(2), 257–269.

LPSSC (The Lifers Public Safety Steering Committee of the State Correctional institution at Graterford, Pennsylvania). (2004). Ending the culture of street crime. *The Prison Journal, 84*(4), 48S–68S.

MacCormick, A. (1931). *The education of adult prisoners: A survey and a program*. New York, NY: National Society of Penal Information.

MacDonald, D. (1995). *Overview of department follow-up research on return rates of participants in major programs 1995*. Albany, NY: New York State Department of Correctional Services.

MacKenzie, D. (1987). Age and adjustment to prison: Interactions with attitudes and anxiety. *Criminal Justice and Behavior, 14*(4), 427–447.

MacKenzie, D., & Goodstein, L. (1985). Long term incarceration impacts and characteristics of long-term offenders: An empirical analysis. *Criminal Justice and Behavior, 12*(4), 395–414.

MacKenzie, D., Robinson, J., & Campbell, C. (1989). Long-term incarceration of female offenders: Prison adjustment and coping. *Criminal Justice and Behavior, 16*(2), 223–238.

Maher, L. (2000). *Sexed work: Gender, race and resistance in a Brooklyn drug market*. New York, NY: Oxford University Press.

Martin, R., Zimmerman, S., & Long, B. (1993). AIDS education in US prisons: A survey of inmate programs. *The Prison Journal, 73*(1), 103–129.

Martinson, R. (1974). What works? Questions and answers about prison reform. *The Public Interest, Spring,* 22–54.

Martinson, R. (1979). New findings, new view: A note of caution regarding sentencing reform. *Hofstral Law Review, 7,* 243–258.

Maruna, S. (2001). *Making good: How ex-convicts reform and rebuild their lives*. Washington, DC: American Psychological Association.

Maruschak, L. (2002). *HIV in prisons, 2000*. Bureau of justice statistics. Washington, DC: US Department of Justice.

Matsueda, R. (1982). Testing control theory and differential association: A causal modeling approach. *American Sociological Review, 47,* 489–504

McCarthy, B. (1980). Inmate mothers: The problems of separation and reintegration. *Journal of Offender Counseling, Services, and Rehabilitation, 4*(3), 199–212.

McClellan, D. (1994). Disparity in the discipline of male and female inmates in Texas prisons. *Women and Criminal Justice, 5*(2), 71–97.

McCollum, S. (1994). Prison college programs. *The Prison Journal, 73*(1), 51–61.

McCord, J. (1986). Instigation and insulation: How families affect antisocial aggression. In D. Olweus, J. Block, & M. Radke-Yarrow (Eds.), *Development of antisocial and prosocial behavior* (pp. 343–357). Orlando, FL: Academic.

McCorkle, R., Miethe, T., & Drass, K. (1995). The roots of prison violence: A test of the deprivation, management, and 'not-so-total' institution models. *Crime and Delinquency, 41*(3), 317–331.

Michalsen, V. (2011). Mothering as a life course transition – Do women go straight for their children? *Journal of Offender Rehabilitation, 50*(6), 349–366.

Miki, J. (1998). *HIV in New York State prisons*. New York, NY: Bureau of HIV/AIDS Epidemiology, New York State Department of Health.

Moffitt, T. E., Caspi, A., Rutter, M., & Silva, P. A. (2001). *Sex differences in antisocial behaviour: Conduct disorder, delinquency and violence in the Dunedin longitudinal study*. Cambridge: Cambridge University Press.

Moyer, I. (1984). Deceptions and realities of life in women's prisons. *The Prison Journal, 64,* 45–56.

Mullings, J., Marquart, J., & Hartley, D. (2003). Exploring the effects of childhood sexual abuse and its impact on HIV/AIDS risk-taking behavior among women prisoners. *The Prison Journal, 83*(4), 442–463.

NCJRS. (2011). *Women and girls in the criminal justice system – Facts and figures*. Retrieved from https://www.ncjrs.gov/spotlight/wgcjs/facts.html.

New York State Department of Health. (2002). *AIDS in New York State: 2001–2002*. Available from http://www.health.state.ny.us/nysdoh/hivaids/aidsny_01/section15.pdf.

Nouwen, H. (1972). *The wounded healer*. New York, NY: Doubleday.

NYSDOCSS (New York State Department of Correctional Services and Supervision) (2012). About DOCCS. Retrieved from: http://www.doccs.ny.gov/, on 8/3/12.

Nuttall, J., Hollmen, L., & Staley, M. (2003). The effect of earning a GED on recidivism rates. *JCE, 54*(3), 90–94.

NYSDOCS (New York State Department of Correctional services) (2008). *Female Offenders: 2005–2006*. New York State Department of Correctional Services.

NYSDOCS (New York State Department of Correctional Services). (2003). *Characteristics of inmates discharged*. Albany, NY: New York State Department of Correctional Services.

NYSDOCS (New York State Department of Correctional Services) (2002). Rates of inmate HIV, AIDS, TB in sharp decline. *DOCS Today,* 10–11.

NYSDOH AIDS Institute. (2008). *Improving health outcomes for HIV positive individuals transitioning from correctional settings to the community*.

O'Brien, E. (1985). Global self-esteem scales: Unidimensional or multidimensional? *Psychological Reports, 57*(2), 383–389.

O'Neil, M. (1990). Correctional higher education: Reduced recidivism? *Journal of Correctional Education, 41*(1), 28–31.

Odem, M. (1995). *Delinquent Daughters: Protecting and policing adolescent female sexuality in the United States, 1885–1920.* North Carolina: UNC Press.

Osborn, S. (1980). Moving home, leaving London and delinquent trends. *British Journal of Criminology, 20*(1), 54–61.

Owen, B. (2004). Women and imprisonment in the United States: The gendered consequences of the U.S. imprisonment binge. In B. Price & N. Sokoloff (Eds.), *The criminal justice system and women: Offenders, prisoners, victims, and workers* (3rd ed., pp. 195–206). New York, NY: McGraw Hill.

Palmer, T. (1995). Programmatic and non-programmatic aspects of successful intervention: New directions for research. *Crime and Delinquency, 41*(1), 100–131.

Pollock, J. (1984). Women will be women: Correctional officers' perceptions of the emotionality of women inmates. *The Prison Journal, 64*(1), 84–91.

Pollock-Byrne, J. (1990). *Women, prison and crime.* California, CA: Brooks/Cole Publishing Company.

Poole, E., & Regoli, R. (1980). Race, institutional rule breaking, and disciplinary response: A study of discretionary making in prison. *Law and Society Review, 14*(4), 931–946.

Propper, A. (1982). Make-believe families and homosexuality among imprisoned girls. *Criminology, 20*(1), 127–138.

Rafter, N. (1989). Gender and justice: The equal protection issue. In *The American Prison: Issues in Research and Policy*, (ed. Goodstein, L., & Mackenzie, D.). New York: Plenum Press, 89–109.

Ramirez, J. (1983). Race and the apprehension of inmate misconduct. *Journal of Criminal Justice, 11*(5), 413–427.

Rankin, J. (1976). Investigating the interrelations among social control variables and conformity. *The Journal of Criminal Law and Criminology, 67*(4), 740–480.

Reed, D., & Reed, E. (2004). Mothers in prison and their children. In B. Price & N. Sokoloff (Eds.), *The criminal justice system and women: Offenders, prisoners, victims, and workers* (3rd ed., pp. 261–273). New York, NY: McGraw Hill.

Reisig, M., Holtfreter, K., & Morash, M. (2002). Social capital among women offenders: Examining the distribution of social networks and resources. *Journal of Contemporary Criminal Justice, 18*(2), 167–187.

Richards, B. (1978). The experience of long term imprisonment: An exploratory investigation. *British Journal of Criminology, 18*(2), 162–169.

Rosenbaum, J. (1987). Social control, gender, and delinquency: An analysis of drug, property and violent offenders. *Justice Quarterly, 4*(1), 117–132.

Rosenberg, M. (1965). *Society and the adolescent self-image.* Princeton, NJ: Princeton University Press.

Roundtree, G., Edwards, D., & Dawson, S. (1982). The effects of education on self-esteem of male prison inmates. *Journal of Correctional Education, 32*(4), 12–18.

Ryan, T., & McCabe, K. (1994). Mandatory versus voluntary prison education and academic achievement. *The Prison Journal, 74*(4), 450–461.

Sampson, R., & Laub, J. (1990). Crime and deviance over the life course: The salience of adult social bonds. *American Sociological Review, 55*(5), 609–627.

Sampson, R., & Laub, J. (1992). Crime and deviance in the life course. *Annual Review of Sociology, 18*, 63–84.

Sampson, R., & Laub, J. (1993). *Crime in the making.* Cambridge, MA: Harvard University Press.

Sampson, R., & Laub, J. (1995). Understanding variability in loves through time: Contributions of life-course criminology. *Studies on Crime and Crime Prevention, 4*(2), 143–158.

Sampson, R., & Laub, J. (1996). Socioeconomic achievement in the life course of disadvantaged men: Military service as a turning point, CIRCA 1940–1965. *American Sociological Review, 61*, 347–367.

Schrag, C. (1944). *Social role types in a prison community*. Master's thesis, University of Washington, Seattle

Shrum, H. (2004). No longer theory: Correctional practices that work. *Journal of Correctional Education, 55*(3), 225–235.

Schulz, D. M. (1995). *From social worker to crime fighter Women in United States municipal policing*. Connecticut: Praeger.

Schumacker, R., Anderson, D., & Anderson, S. (1990). Vocational and academic indicators of parole success. *Journal of Correctional Education, 41*(1), 8–13.

Schur, E. M. (1984). *Labeling women deviant gender, stigma and social control*. New York, NY: Random House.

Sepsi, V. (1974). Girl recidivists. *Journal of Research in Crime and Delinquency, 11*(1), 70–79.

Shover, N., Norland, S., James, J., & Thornton, W. (1979). Gender roles and Delinquency. *Social Forces, 58*(1), 162–175.

Smart, C. (1976). *Women, crime, and criminology: A feminist critique*. London: Routledge & Kegan Paul Ltd.

Smith, D., & Paternoster, R. (1987). The gender gap in theories of deviance: Issues and evidence. *Journal of Research in Crime and Delinquency, 24*(2), 140–172.

Smith, L., & Silverman, M. (1994). Functional literacy education for jail inmates: An examination of the Hillsborough County Jail education program. *The Prison Journal, 74*(4), 414–431.

Snell, T., & Morton, D. (1994). *Women in prison: Survey of state inmates prison inmates, 1991*. Bureau of justice statistics special report. Washington, DC: US Department of Justice.

Sommers, I., Baskin, D., & Fagan, J. (1994). Getting out of the life: Crime desistance by female street offenders. *Deviant Behavior, 15*(2), 125–149.

Staley, M. (2001). *Follow-up study of offenders who earned GEDs while incarcerated in DOCS*. New York State Department of Correctional Services.

Staley, M. (2003). *Female offenders: 2001–2002*. Albany, NY: New York State Department of Correctional Services.

Steffensmeier, D., & Allan, E. (1996). Gender and crime: Toward a gendered theory of female offending. *Annual Review of Sociology, 22*, 459–487.

Stephan, J. (1989). *Prison rule violators*. Bureau of justice statistics special report. Washington DC: US Department of Justice

Sternberg, S. (2004) HIV infection rates appear to be rising in USA. *USA Today*. Available from http://www.usatoday.com/news/health/2003-02-11-hiv-rates-rising_x.htm.

Suter, J., Byrne, M., Byrne, S., Howells, K., & Day, A. (2002). Anger in prisoners: Women are different from men. *Personality and Individual Differences, 32*(6), 1087–1100.

Sutherland, E. (1949). *White Collar Crime*. New York: Holt, Rinehart & Winston.

Syed, F., & Blanchette, K. (2000a). *Results of an evaluation of the peer support program at Joliette Institution for Women*. Research Branch: Correctional Service of Canada.

Syed, F., & Blanchette, K. (2000b). *Results of an evaluation of the peer support program at Grand Valley institution for Women*. Research Branch: Correctional Service of Canada.

Sykes, G. (1958). *The society of captives: A study of maximum security prisons*. Princeton, NJ: Princeton University Press.

Sykes, G., & Messinger, S. (1960). Inmate social systems. In R. Cloward (Ed.), *Theoretical studies in social organization of the prison* (pp. 5–19). New York, NY: Social Science Research Council.

Taylor, J. (1992). Post-secondary correctional education: An evaluation of effectiveness and efficiency. *Journal of Correctional Education, 43*(3), 132–141.

Taylor, M. (1993). Pell grants for prisoners. *The Nation, 256*, 88–91.

Tewksbury, R. (1994). Literacy programming for jail inmates: Reflections and recommendations from one program. *The Prison Journal, 74*(4), 398–413.

Tewksbury, R., & Vito, G. (1994). Improving the educational skills of jail inmates: Preliminary program findings. *Federal Probation, LVIII*(2), 55–59.

Tischler, C., & Marquart, J. (1989). Analysis of disciplinary infraction rates among female and male inmates. *Journal of Criminal Justice, 17*(6), 507–513.

Toch, H., & Adams, K. (1986). Pathology and disruptiveness among prison inmates. *Journal of Research in Crime and Delinquency, 23*(1), 7–21.

Toch, H., & Grant, D. (1989). Noncoping and maladaptation in confinement. In L. Goodstein & D. Mackenzie (Eds.), *The American prison: Issues in research and policy*. New York, NY: Plenum.

Tootoonchi, A. (1993). College education in prisons: The inmates' perspectives. *Federal Probation, LVII*(4), 34–40.

Torstensson, M. (1990). Female delinquents in a birth cohort: Tests of some aspects of control theory. *Journal of Quantitative Criminology, 6*(1), 101–115.

Travis, J. (2002). Invisible punishment: An instrument of social exclusion. In M. Mauer & M. Chesney-Lind (Eds.), *Invisible Punishment: The collateral consequence of mass imprisonment* (pp. 15–36). New York, NY: New Press.

Travis, J., Solomon, A. L., & Waul, M. (2001). *When prisoners come home: The dimensions and consequences of prisoner reentry*. Washington, DC: Urban Institute/Justice Policy Center. Retrieved from http://www.urban.org/pdfs/from_prison_to_home.pdf.

Trites, R., & Fiedorowicz, C. (1991). An effective reading program for inmates. *American Jails, V*(3), 73–78.

United States Conference of Mayors. (1995). HIV prevention education in city/county jails. *AIDS Information Exchange, 12*(4), 1–3.

Van Voorhis, P. (1987). Correctional effectiveness: The high cost of ignoring success. *Federal Probation, LI*(1), 56–62.

Welch, M. (1996). *Corrections: A critical approach*. New York, NY: McGraw-Hall.

Wheeler, S. (1961). Socialization in correctional communities. *American Sociological Review, 26*(5), 694–712.

Wiatrowski, M., Griswold, D., & Roberts, M. (1981). Social control theory and delinquency. *American Sociological Review, 46*, 525–541.

Wolf, S., Freinek, W., & Shaffer, J. (1966). Frequency and severity of rule infractions as criteria of prison maladjustment. *Journal of Clinical Psychology, 22*(2), 244–248.

Wolfgang, M. (1961). Quantitative analysis of adjustment to the prison community. *The Journal of Criminal Law, Criminology, and Police Science, 51*(6), 607–618.

Wolfgang, M. E., Figilio, R. M., & Sellin, T. (1972). *Delinquency in a birth cohort*. Chicago: University of Chicago Press.

Women in Prison Project. (2009). *Women in prison fact sheet*. Retrieved from http://www.correction-alassociation.org/publications/download/wipp/factsheets/Wome_in_Prison Fact Sheet 2009 FINAL.pdf.

Worthen, M. (2011). Gender differences in parent–child bonding: Implications for understanding the gender gap in delinquency. *Journal of Crime and Justice, 34*(1), 3–23.

Wright, K. (1999). A study of individual, environmental, and interactive effects in explaining adjustment to prison. *Justice Quarterly, 8*(2), 217–242.

Yarbo, K. (1996). Saving money or wasting minds? *Corrections Today, 12*(14), 16.

Yeager, M. (2003a). Life-course study of released prisoners suggests importance of employment for offender reintegration and community safety. *Offender Programs Report, 7*(2), 27–32.

Yeager, M. (2003b). A review of the literature on employment, marriage, and reoffending. *Offender Programs Reports, 7*(2), 29–31.

Index

K. Collica, *Female Prisoners, AIDS, and Peer Programs: How Female
Offenders Transform Their Lives*, SpringerBriefs in Psychology,
DOI 10.1007/978-1-4614-5110-5, © The Author 2013